T0073087

Prostasin in Human Health and Disease

Li-Mei Chen

University of Central Florida, USA

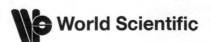

NEW JERSEY · LONDON · SINGAPORE · BEIJING · SHANGHAI · HONG KONG · TAIPEI · CHENNAI · TOKYO

Published by

World Scientific Publishing Co. Pte. Ltd.

5 Toh Tuck Link, Singapore 596224

USA office: 27 Warren Street, Suite 401-402, Hackensack, NJ 07601

UK office: 57 Shelton Street, Covent Garden, London WC2H 9HE

Library of Congress Cataloging-in-Publication Data

Names: Chen, Li-Mei, author.

Title: Prostasin in human health and disease / Li-Mei Chen.

Description: New Jersey : World Scientific, [2023] | Includes bibliographical references and index.

Identifiers: LCCN 2022054085 | ISBN 9789811268144 (hardcover) |

ISBN 9789811268151 (ebook for institutions) |

ISBN 9789811268168 (ebook other for individuals)

Subjects: MESH: Serine Endopeptidases

Classification: LCC QP609.S47 | NLM QU 136 | DDC 572/.76--dc23/eng/20230201

LC record available at https://lccn.loc.gov/2022054085

British Library Cataloguing-in-Publication Data

A catalogue record for this book is available from the British Library.

For any available supplementary material, please visit
https://www.worldscientific.com/worldscibooks/10.1142/13195#t=suppl

Desk Editor: Vanessa Quek ZhiQin

Typeset by Stallion Press
Email: enquiries@stallionpress.com

Contents

Prologue   vii
Editorial Comment   xi

Chapter 1   The Serine Proteases — A Brief Overview   1

Chapter 2   The Membrane Serine Proteases — Classification
             and Overview   11

Chapter 3   Prostasin Serine Protease — 30 Years of
             Discoveries   21

Chapter 4   The Basic Molecular Information on Prostasin   35

Chapter 5   The Structure, the Function, and the Regulation   49

Chapter 6   The Roles in Physiology and Pathophysiology —
             An Overview   63

Chapter 7   Prostasin in the Kidney — Regulating the
             ENaC Activity   73

Chapter 8   Prostasin in the Airways   85

Chapter 9   Prostasin in the Intestinal Tract   99

Chapter 10   Prostasin in the Skin   111

Chapter 11   Prostasin in the Reproductive Organs   121

Chapter 12   Prostasin in Inflammation and Infection   133

Chapter 13   Prostasin in Other Organs   145

Chapter 14   Prostasin in Cancer   157

Chapter 15   Prostasin Substrates, Regulators, and Inhibitors   181

Chapter 16   Prostasin as a Biomarker, a Drug Target, and in
                    Therapeutic Development   203

Epilogue   231
Index   235

Prologue

The human prostasin was discovered almost 30 years ago simply as a trypsin-like serine protease in the seminal plasma, followed by the molecular cloning of its cDNA and gene. A few years later, an epithelial sodium channel (ENaC) activator, named xCAP1, was discovered in Xenopus and proposed to be the orthologue of the human prostasin based on their high amino acid sequence similarities. Subsequently, the mouse and rat homologues of xCAP1 were identified and named as mCAP1 and rCAP1, respectively, based on sequence as well as functional similarities, while the search for the xCAP1 functional orthologue in human airway tissues yielded prostasin. In the ensuing years, research on prostasin by laboratories around the world has built a vast repertoire of knowledge and information on its structure, function, and genetics, as well as potential links to human health and disease. Prostasin is a multi-functional serine protease anchored extracellularly to the surface plasma membrane via glycosylated and phosphorylated lipids, involved in the regulation of sodium transport via the ENaC, of epithelial permeability via the cell-cell junction proteins, of outside-in cellular signaling pathway activation via the tyrosine kinase receptors (RTK) and protease-activated receptor-2 (PAR-2). Prostasin is implicated in physiological and pathological manifestations of a broad range of cellular programs, including proliferation, migration, invasion, and the epithelial-to-mesenchymal transition (EMT). Most important, prostasin is recognized as a marker in the maturation of the epithelium.

Water and oxygen are the two most essential matters of life. Oxygen carried by the red blood cells goes everywhere in the body, driven by the blood flow. Water constitutes 70% of the body weight. The water inside the body is preserved by the skin, lung, kidney, and colon, by the cells in the epithelium lining all body parts, externally and internally. Water can go into cells along with the active Na^+ reabsorption involving the ENaC or to the intercellular and interstitial spaces by the paracellular movement involving the tight junction apparatus. The homeostasis of water and Na^+ at the proper volume and pressure in a body is essential to a healthy life. As an ENaC activator and a regulator of the cellular tight junctions, prostasin is integral to the maintenance of the water and Na^+ homeostasis. However, these functions appear dispensable in some tissues, suggesting that compensatory mechanisms may be at play. Studies have also shown that prostasin has other potentially highly important functions independent of its role as an activator of the ENaC.

An absence of prostasin from the whole body via a germline gene knockout is embryonic lethal to mice, and the defects are manifested early with insufficient placental development. Formation of the placenta is a controlled process of immune tolerance and inflammation, in which cell proliferation, invasion, immune surveillance, and cytokine production are managed in a time- and space-specific manner. This is a good example of investigating the prostasin functions in pathophysiological conditions, *in vivo* or with *in vitro* cell models. Whereas under the normal and basic physiological conditions there is not a good phenotypic outcome to show what prostasin is doing. We will see such concepts and approaches play out in the key investigations on the biological functions of prostasin, such as ENaC activation.

The uniqueness of the prostasin serine protease is its membrane anchorage via a glycosylphosphatidylinositol (GPI) moiety. This anchorage exposes the entire prostasin molecule on the outside cell surface and makes prostasin a good candidate as a biomarker or drug target when its roles in a disease condition is established. With this anchorage, prostasin can be released by epithelial cells in the extracellular vesicles known as the exosomes, as an active proteolytic enzyme. This feature could be exploited as a method of delivery if prostasin is used as a potential therapeutic agent for conditions with a prostasin deficiency.

It is estimated that humans have 699 proteases, among them 178 are serine proteases and among them 138 belong to the S1 protease family. Chymotrypsin and trypsin were the first mammalian serine proteases to be isolated and studied, extensively, owing to their abundance in the bovine pancreas and the relative ease of purification. The studies on trypsin date back to Wilhelm Kühne in 1876 when it was first discovered and isolated, but new discoveries on this prototypic serine protease continue to be made today, with much more sophistication and relevance to health and disease, and application.

Prostasin was discovered in the mid-1990's but owing to the fast pace in technological advancements, a great deal has already been learned about its functions in many aspects such as electrolyte homeostasis, skin integrity, receptor tyrosine kinase regulation, immunity, inflammation, and cancer development and progression. In this book, we will highlight the key findings and will also present the challenges and unsolved problems that the prostasin research community has experienced and identified.

Editorial Comment

The human body has an estimated 37 trillion cells on average, and they form the various organs and tissues with more than 200 histologically distinguishable cell types. All the cells originated from one single fertilized egg, endowed with a diploid genome from the parental gametic haploid cells, a sperm and an egg. In the journey from 1 to 37 trillion, the cells divide via mitosis and differentiate to become specialized in their roles and functions, maintained in a homeostasis but dynamically changing to adapt to the changes in the environments — of the body and of the cells. Along the way, the developing embryo invaginates and folds into a layered left-right symmetry. The three layers, the endoderm, the mesoderm, and the ectoderm morph into the body's anatomical systems. Most of the cells share the basic structure with a nucleus and the various subcellular compartments connected or communicating with one another via the lipid bilayer membrane. At the molecular level, in each cell, the diploid DNA genome has 3 billion base pairs (bp) of genetic information in each haploid, carried by 23 pairs of chromosomes with 22 autosomes and sex chromosomes of either XX or XY. By the Central Dogma of life, the protein-coding genes can be transcribed to transfer the genetic information to the messenger RNA, which can be translated to produce polypeptides that eventually fold into proteins with three-dimensional structures. The biological functions of the proteins are endowed by their biological structures and both can change as a result of changes in the cell's environment. There are upwards of 25,000 protein-coding genes in the human genome, which can undergo changes too, as a result of perpetuated replicative errors or chemical damages induced by an external agent, such as radiation. The differentiation or specialization of cells in the various organs and tissues of the body is marked by a unique cellular molecular landscape of the proteins and other macromolecules that are produced by the proteins. Some genes that produce proteins to maintain the basic level of existence for the cells are expressed all the time, but not all of the genes are expressed in all the cells all the time, and not all of the genes are expressed in any single cells all the time or at any time. The molecular landscape of a specific cell type also changes dynamically with the changes in the cell's environment. Since all cells in a body contain the same genome with the same genetic information, barring yet accepting the errors and mutations accumulated in the course of development, the selective expression of genes in the differentiated and specialized cells is achieved by controlling gene expression switches. These are the chemical modifications of the genomic DNA such as cytosine methylation and of the chromatin components such as histone tail acetylation. Some cells maintain an undifferentiated state, the stemness, and are the sources for replenishment of lost or damaged cells. The germ cells in the reproductive system undergo a reductive division known as meiosis and make the haploid sperm and eggs for the next cycle of life.

Such is the natural wonder of the human body and it is entirely unjust to reduce it to one paragraph of technical language as above. It is, however, a background needed for painting the best picture for our main character of this book, the prostasin serine protease. We will see that this unique and versatile protein plays a role in so many physiological and pathophysiological processes all throughout the entire cycle of human life, from embryonic development to reproduction. To say that prostasin is literally everywhere and in every moment is not a gross overstatement. Prostasin has an essential role in embryonic development as shown by the lethality in embryo of a homozygous double gene knockout in mice. In the epithelium, the best characterized biochemical function of the prostasin serine protease is the proteolytic activation of the epithelial sodium channel, but a loss of prostasin expression is associated with high-grade epithelial tumors, invasion, and metastasis. Whereas in the ovaries, an over-expression of prostasin is associated with tumorigenesis. Perhaps due to prostasin's essential role in a cellular molecular landscape where it is expressed, gene mutations at the genomic DNA level have not been documented in many cases. The regulation of prostasin gene expression is achieved at the epigenetic level by DNA and chromatin modifications, and at the transcription level by factors that are involved in the early embryonic development, such as SNAIL and SLUG. Prostasin is anchored to the cell membrane by a lipid tail, and transcription factors such as the sterol-response element-binding proteins can regulate prostasin expression. The latter themselves sense the changes of cholesterol levels in the cell and in the membrane. These are a few highlights of our main character, prostasin. We will properly introduce and address the current knowledge and remaining questions on prostasin in the chapters.

By Karl X. Chai, Ph.D.
University of Central Florida
College of Medicine

Chapter 1

The Serine Proteases — A Brief Overview

Proteases are enzymes found in all organisms including eukaryotes, prokaryotes, and viruses, and are needed to catalyze the protein peptide bond hydrolysis, a process known as proteolysis. Proteases that cleave the polypeptide chain internally are endopeptidases while those that cleave from the amino- or carboxyl-terminus of a polypeptide chain are exopeptidases. Based on the catalytic mechanism, proteases can be divided into six groups, i.e., aspartic proteases, cysteine proteases, metalloproteases, serine proteases, threonine proteases[1], and the recently recognized glutamic proteases[2].

These different classes of protease mediate various cellular processes intracellularly and extracellularly. Aspartic proteases, such as cathepsin D, degrade the endocytosed proteins in the lysosomes[3,4]. Cysteine proteases, such as caspases, working intracellularly in a cascade, are responsible for the proteolysis in apoptosis[5,6]. Metalloproteinases (MMPs), such as MMP2 and MMP9, target substrates in the extracellular matrix[7,8]. Threonine proteases, such as the catalytic subunits of the proteasome complex, degrade damaged or ill-folded proteins[9,10].

Serine proteases have a broad spectrum of functions depending on their structure. Most of them belong to the S1 family (the chymotrypsin fold) in the PA clan (Proteases of mixed nucleophile, superfamily A). As named, serine proteases use a serine side chain at the active site to form the requisite oxyanion to carry out the nucleophilic attack on the peptide bond. Along with two other amino acid residues, a histidine as the base for accepting the hydrogen from the serine –OH group or the water –OH group and an aspartate to assist the histidine, the three amino acid residues constitute the catalytic triad in a charge relay system

1

in the catalytic cleavage of a peptide bond. The three amino acid residues of the catalytic triad are identified in a linear sequence as histidine57, aspartate102, and serine195 (with the chymotrypsin numbering), but form a catalytic pocket (the S1 pocket) upon folding of the protease's polypeptide into the proper three-dimensional structure. The tertiary structure after the peptide folding consists of two beta-barrel domains aligned at a right angle with each other, and forms the active site where the catalytic action takes place.

The proteolytic reaction catalyzed by a serine protease begins with the deprotonation of the hydroxyl group of the active-site serine, with the imidazole of the active-site histidine serving as the proton acceptor (Figure 1-1).

The active-site aspartate assists the histidine in the deprotonation but it is not essential for the proteolytic action. Thus, some serine proteases contain a catalytic diad with only the serine and the histidine. The serine oxyanion attacks the carbon of the carbonyl group in the peptide bond to be cleaved, known as the scissile bond. This attack is called a nucleophilic attack and a tetrahedral complex is presumed to form between the active-site serine and the carbon of the scissile bond. Cleavage of the scissile bond occurs when its nitrogen accepts the proton held by the active-site histidine, with the formation of an acyl-enzyme intermediate between the amino-terminal portion of the substrate peptide and the active-site serine and the leaving of the carboxyl-terminal portion. The scissile peptide bond is already cleaved at this moment, but no water is involved yet. The serine protease enzyme is reverted to the starting form with another nucleophilic attack, this time with a water molecule undergoing deprotonation by the active-site histidine and the resulting oxyanion from the water molecule forming a tetrahedral complex with the acyl-enzyme complex via the carbon in the carbonyl group. The oxygen of the active-site serine then accepts the water molecule's proton held by the histidine, kicking off the amino-terminal portion of the substrate peptide, completing the cleavage and the reversion of the enzyme itself. The proteolysis catalyzed by a serine protease is technically a hydrolysis only when viewed as a whole process involving the two nucleophilic attack steps. The net effect shows a water molecule being split and given to the two new termini from the cleaved scissile peptide bond.

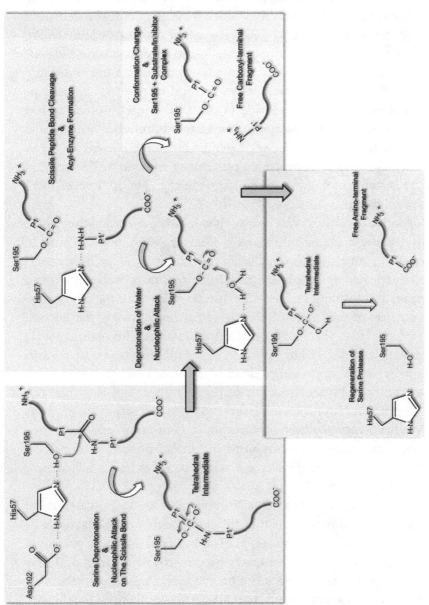

Figure 1-1. Simplified serine protease reaction mechanism. The suicide inhibitor/substrate step if the amino-terminal fragment fails to dissociate is shaded sky blue.

Similar to serine proteases, proteases in the other groups also use nucleophilic attacks as the mechanism of cleaving the substrate peptide bond. For example, the cysteine proteases use the deprotonated thiol group, whereas the metalloproteases use either a glutamate side chain, or water to carry out this action. Only in the latter case, the cleavage of the substrate peptide is a true hydrolysis because a water molecule is literally split by the enzyme's active site and inserted via a nucleophilic attack into the scissile peptide bond. In the reaction mechanism of serine proteases, the cleavage of the scissile bond does not actually involve a water molecule per se. A water molecule is used to break apart the acyl-enzyme complex to return the enzyme to the original form. This step is not always executed as in the case of "irreversible" protease inhibitors.

For serine proteases, a class of such inhibitors are called "serpins", literally "serine protease inhibitors". They are described as "suicide substrates" because the scissile bond in the inhibitor polypeptide can be cleaved by the first nucleophilic attack from a serine protease, involving the serine, and forming the acyl-enzyme complex with the amino-terminal portion of the inhibitor. A conformational change that ensues, however, prevents the second nucleophilic attack involving water, rendering the amino-terminal portion of the inhibitor to be stuck onto the enzyme. A stable covalent complex is formed between the serine protease and the "stuck" portion of the inhibitor. For example, the neurotrophic protein protease nexin-1 (PN-1) is a serpin. It binds to the serine protease prostasin to form a covalent complex which contains both an inactive prostasin and the "stuck" portion of the PN-1 molecule[11,12]. The fate of the serpin-enzyme complex (SEC) is clearance via the SEC receptors.

In addition to the "irreversible" inhibitors of serine proteases, there are "reversible" inhibitors, such as the hepatocyte growth factor activator (HGFA) inhibitors 1 and 2, HAI-1 and HAI-2. These reversible inhibitors interact with the proteases by non-covalent forces and may compete with the substrate for the protease active site (competitive), bind to the protease after substrate binding (uncompetitive), or induce an allosteric conformation change to the protease (non-competitive). The reversible nature of such inhibitors would allow for them to serve as a reservoir of the active enzyme, for example, the transmembrane HAI-1 binds to active HGFA to sequester the latter at the cell surface[13].

The amino acid residue at the bottom of the S1 pocket determines the specificity of the enzyme. Only the correct and specific scissile bond of a substrate can be inserted into the active site of the enzyme upon substrate binding to the enzyme. For example, trypsin has aspartate189 at the bottom of the S1 pocket. This negatively charged amino acid residue attracts and stabilizes the positively charged side chain of arginine or lysine on the amino-terminal side of the scissile amide bond of a substrate, known as the P1 position. Similar to trypsin, prostasin has aspartate232 at the bottom of the S1 pocket, and it confers the specificity and serves as the attractant for substrates having lysine or arginine in the P1 position. Therefore, prostasin is a trypsin-like serine protease. Chymotrypsin, on the other hand, has serine189 at the bottom of the S1 pocket, preferring tyrosine, phenylalanine, and tryptophan at the P1 position of substrates. The "substrate specificity" of a serine protease is almost never absolute. The more stringent enzymes such as prostasin, does not cleave after every arginine or lysine, in one sense of the term "limited proteolysis". The specificity is also dependent on the neighboring residues of the scissile bond, but these do allow some degrees of overlap and an enzyme may have more than one cutting site in one substrate or have more than one substrate peptide. Enzymes with less stringent substrate requirements such as the digestive serine protease trypsin, would cleave after every arginine or lysine in one or any substrate, making it the protease of choice for peptide mapping in the initial years of protein biochemistry to today in modern techniques such as matrix-assisted laser desorption/ionization-time of flight (MALDI-TOF) mass spectrometry (MS).

Due to the "destructive" nature of their functions, whether a serine protease has a broad substrate spectrum like the digestive enzymes or is highly specific for limited proteolysis like prostasin, the proteolysis must be controlled to protect the body's homeostasis. So, when and how are serine proteases called upon for action, and when and how is the proteolytic action controlled? Gene expression up-regulation in response to external stimuli to a system or a tissue/cell type is the basic molecular genetic mechanism to increase the production. The mobilized protease production can also be regulated during protein translation and transport, or post-translationally involving chemical modifications or co-factors. Maintaining a pool of proteases at the post-translational level in an inactive form is quite advantageous when a protease may be called upon for a more immediate action. On one hand, this can be achieved with two mechanisms, precursors and reversible inhibitors, e.g., HAI-1. On the other hand, the irreversible protease inhibitors, i.e., serpins, serve to permanently remove the proteases when their removal is necessary.

Most serine proteases are synthesized as precursors, known as zymogens, and enter the secretory pathway. The amino-terminal pro-peptides are cleaved to generate the active enzymes, but the cleaved pro-peptides could still be bound via disulfide bonds to the peptidase domains. For example, the pro-protein of prostasin is cleaved between arginine12 (R44 when the pre-peptide is included) and isoleucine13 to produce a light chain and a heavy chain, and the two chains are disulfide-linked[14,15]. The benefit of proteases, including serine proteases to be ever present as zymogens, is the ability for an immediate participation in a physiological event that requires their actions when production via gene expression does not meet the requirement of urgency. The proenzymes are not entirely inactive but the conformation of the enzymes in the zymogen form does not allow for the most efficient cleavage of substrates, which can be the zymogen themselves[16].

The physiological importance of zymogen activation and mobilization of additional enzymes cannot be better demonstrated by the trypsin-like serine proteases in the blood coagulation cascade[17] (Figure 1-2).

The serine protease blood coagulation Factor VII is the first to be activated during tissue injury, known as the extrinsic pathway. In the intrinsic pathway, the serine protease Factor XII is the first to be activated upon exposure to the damaged blood vessel surface. The surface binding of Factor XII can induce a conformational change and result in its autoactivation, via cleavage at Arg353–Val354, producing the active Factor XIIa, at 80-kDa with a heavy and a light chain held by a disulfide bond. The now activated Factor XIIa can go on to activate more Factor XII zymogen. The surface binding also serves as a means of concentrating the zymogen to the site of action. The active Factor

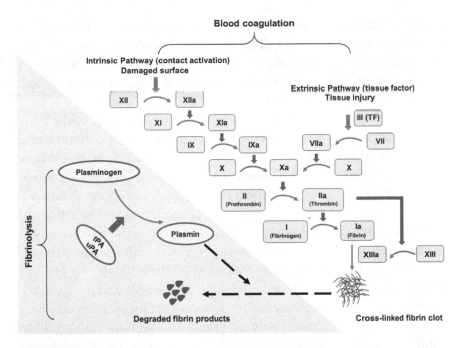

Figure 1-2. Simplified blood coagulation cascade and fibrinolysis. Green arrows: initial triggers, brown arrows: activating proteins, blue arrows: activating reactions, dotted lines: cutting and degrading reactions.

XIIa activates Factor XI to XIa in the next step, then the activation event passes a cascade of zymogen activation via Factors IX and X, prothrombin and finally to the end point of fibrinogen proteolytic processing and the formation of cross-linked fibrin clots. Among all participating clotting factors, many are serine proteases, while tissue factor (Factor III), Factor V, Factor VIII are glycoproteins working as co-factors of serine proteases. Factor XIII is a transglutaminase. The extrinsic and intrinsic pathways merge at the point of Factor X activation before the activation of prothrombin to thrombin by Xa.

This chain reaction ensures an amplification of the initial signal to the end biological function, but the cascade relay can be broken at any point along the chain reaction, for example, as the result of a mutation in an enzyme of the proteolytic activation cascade. If the clotting cascade is interrupted, as in the cases of Factor VIII deficiency (hemophilia A),

Factor IX deficiency (hemophilia B), or Factor XI deficiency (hemophilia C), a longer bleeding time will be the clinical outcome which is detrimental and could be life threatening due to the loss of a large volume of blood. Identification and characterization of such "breaking points" provide opportunities for drug intervention of the disease.

Whereas blood coagulation leading to hemostasis is vital to the body in the event of an injury to prevent the loss of blood, the counteracting process of fibrinolysis is equally important to maintain the blood flow by clearing intrinsic clots[18]. This is achieved also by proteolytic enzymes, with plasmin being the direct fibrin-cleaving serine protease. Plasmin is activated by proteolysis of its zymogen, plasminogen, via the actions of serine proteases tissue plasminogen activator (tPA) and urokinase-type plasminogen activator (uPA). A disruption of the fibrinolysis pathway may result in the pathological condition of thrombosis. To prevent thrombosis or abnormal bleeding[19], both fibrinolysis and hemostasis/ coagulation must be regulated, and an important mechanism is by way of enzyme-specific serine protease inhibitors, such as antithrombin (inhibiting Factor Xa and thrombin), heparin cofactor II (inhibiting thrombin), α1-antitrypsin (inhibiting thrombin and plasmin), protein C inhibitor (broad spectrum), α2-antiplasmin, and plasminogen activator inhibitor-1.

In addition to blood coagulation and fibrinolysis, in humans, proteolytic enzymes perform many essential biological functions in a life cycle including reproduction and embryonic development, food digestion, inflammation, apoptosis, and immunity. Most important in the involvement of proteases are the control and regulation of their proteolytic activities. Only the right enzyme(s) must be mobilized for the right physiological event, via gene expression up-regulation or release/activation from an active enzyme or zymogen pool. Only the right substrate(s) must be cleaved by the mobilized enzyme(s), via the discrimination by the enzyme active site pocket. And in the end, the enzyme(s) must be inhibited either reversibly or irreversibly. The fine and delicate balance between these counteracting forces and factors will be a key focus of our discussion throughout this book on the plethora of functions of the prostasin serine protease.

References

1. Barrett AJ, Rawlings ND, Salvesen G, Woessner JF (2013). Introduction. In *Handbook of Proteolytic Enzymes (Third Edition)*, Rawlings ND, Salvesen G (eds.), Academic Press, li–liv.
2. Fujinaga M, Cherney MM, Oyama H, Oda K, James MN (2004). The molecular structure and catalytic mechanism of a novel carboxyl peptidase from Scytalidium lignicolum. *Proc Natl Acad Sci USA.* 101(10):3364–3369.
3. Szecsi PB (1992). The aspartic proteases. *Scand J Clin Lab Invest Suppl.* 210:5–22.
4. Fusek M, Mares M, Vetvicka V (2012). Chapter 8 — Cathepsin D. In *Handbook of Proteolytic Enzymes (Third Edition)*, Rawlings ND, Salvesen G (eds.), Academic Press, 54–63.
5. Chapman HA, Riese RJ, Shi GP (1997). Emerging roles for cysteine proteases in human biology. *Annu Rev Physiol.* 59:63–88.
6. Creagh EM (2014). Caspase crosstalk: Integration of apoptotic and innate immune signalling pathways. *Trends Immunol.* 35(12):631–640.
7. Rawlings ND, Barrett AJ (1995). Evolutionary families of metallopeptidases. *Methods Enzymol.* 248:183–228.
8. Nagase H, Woessner JF (1999). Matrix metalloproteinases. *J Biol Chem.* 274(31):21491–21494.
9. Rechsteiner M (2013). Proteasomes, Overview. In *Encyclopedia of Biological Chemistry (Second Edition)*, Lennarz WJ, Lane MD (eds.), Academic Press, 590–594.
10. Huber EM, Heinemeyer W, Li X, Arendt CS, Hochstrasser M, Groll M (2016). A unified mechanism for proteolysis and autocatalytic activation in the 20S proteasome. *Nat Commun.* 7:10900.
11. Chen LM, Skinner ML, Kauffman SW, Chao J, Chao L, Thaler CD, Chai KX (2001). Prostasin is a glycosylphosphatidylinositol-anchored active serine protease. *J Biol Chem.* 276(24):21434–21442.
12. Chen LM, Zhang X, Chai KX (2004). Regulation of prostasin expression and function in the prostate. *Prostate.* 59(1):1–12.
13. Kataoka H, Shimomura T, Kawaguchi T, Hamasuna R, Itoh H, Kitamura N, Miyazawa K, Koono M (2000). Hepatocyte growth factor activator inhibitor type 1 is a specific cell surface binding protein of hepatocyte growth factor activator (HGFA) and regulates HGFA activity in the pericellular microenvironment. *J Biol Chem.* 275(51):40453–40462.

14. Yu JX, Chao L, Chao J (1994). Prostasin is a novel human serine proteinase from seminal fluid. Purification, tissue distribution, and localization in prostate gland. *J Biol Chem.* 269(29):18843–18848.
15. Yu JX, Chao L, Chao J (1995). Molecular cloning, tissue-specific expression, and cellular localization of human prostasin mRNA. *J Biol Chem.* 270(22):13483–13489.
16. Gohara DW, Di Cera E (2011). Allostery in trypsin-like proteases suggests new therapeutic strategies. *Trends Biotechnol.* 29(11):577–585.
17. Palta S, Saroa R, Palta A (2014). Overview of the coagulation system. *Indian J Anaesth.* 58(5):515–523.
18. Chapin JC, Hajjar KA (2015). Fibrinolysis and the control of blood coagulation. *Blood Rev.* 29(1):17–24.
19. Bianchini EP, Auditeau C, Razanakolona M, Vasse M, Borgel D (2021). Serpins in hemostasis as therapeutic targets for bleeding or thrombotic disorders. *Front Cardiovasc Med.* 7:622778.

Chapter 2

The Membrane Serine Proteases — Classification and Overview

"A cell is regarded as the true biological atom", "As a cell the organism commences", "Life is the dynamical condition of the organism"[1]. A cell in a multicellular organism has to interact with its neighboring cells in a solid tissue such as the liver, as well as in a fluid tissue such as the blood. The structure and topology of the lipid bilayer plasma membrane of a cell is in a continuum with the inner membranous structures via vesicular trafficking. The membrane is dynamically changing in shape and composition to adapt to the cell's structural needs, driven by the dynamic cytoskeleton attached to the inner leaflet of the cell membrane. Integral membrane proteins traverse across and may have functional domains on both sides of the membrane, and peripheral membrane proteins congregate at the membrane on both sides to reach a critical concentration and initiate biochemical reactions.

Cell-cell communications keep the integrity of the tissue in check in normal physiology and are essential for the proper repair of tissue damage. In the blood, Cluster of Differentiation 40 (CD40) ligand (CD40L) found on the T helper cells can interact with the CD40 receptor on activated B cells to initiate functional changes in the B cells[2]. In a solid tissue, a phenomenon called "contact inhibition", first described in the 1950's[3] and referring to the "monolayering" of fibroblast cells grown *in vitro* in a tissue culture dish, has been investigated ever since with the intent of identifying the "contact inhibitors". The term was initially used strictly on the cessation of cell movement and proliferation once the cells grow to form a perfect monolayer in the dish. Cells

11

would not grow on top of one another, and the inhibition of movement and proliferation is triggered by the cell-cell contact. The term has a broader meaning now and not the least would imply the cessation of DNA replication as well. This would make sense as the cessation of proliferation is mechanistically executed at the molecular level.

Clearly, membrane proteins are the best and most reasonable candidates to play the role of "contact inhibitors". One example of contact inhibition in the physiological context *in vivo* is epithelial wound healing, though herein a more complex set of cells must orchestrate in the tissue context to complete the contact inhibition. Both *in vitro* and *in vivo*, a loss of contact inhibition is thus regarded as a hallmark of cancer.

Most serine proteases are secreted to the outside of the cell as soluble proteins, but a number of membrane-bound extracellular serine proteases were discovered in the past 30 or so years, such as hepsin, matriptase, and prostasin. Currently, there are three known types of membrane anchorage for serine proteases (Figure 2-1).

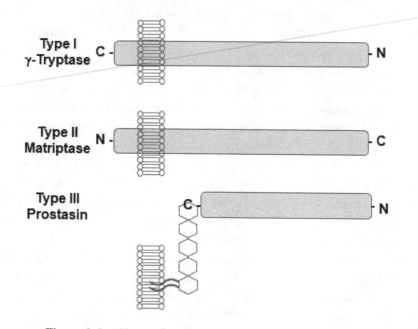

Figure 2-1. Types of membrane serine proteases (examples).

Type I transmembrane serine proteases are anchored to the plasma membrane by a carboxyl-terminal transmembrane domain with the amino terminus on the outside of the cell, e.g., gamma-tryptase[4]. Type II transmembrane serine proteases are anchored to the plasma membrane via an amino-terminal transmembrane domain with the carboxyl terminus on the outside of the cell, e.g., hepsin and matriptase[5-8]. Alternatively (or type III), the anchorage of the serine protease peptide is not directly on the membrane, but through a lipid moiety, a glycosylphosphatidylinositol (GPI) attached to the carboxyl-terminus of the serine proteases, e.g., prostasin[9,10]. The GPI provides the anchor to the plasma membrane while the entire serine protease peptide is on the outside of the cell.

Type I transmembrane proteins traverse the endoplasmic reticulum membrane one time during biosynthesis, whereas Type II transmembrane proteins do so twice, ending with their carboxyl-terminus presented on the outside of the plasma membrane. Whereas the serine proteases of the blood coagulation cascade are present in a soluble environment and the activation is triggered by a concentrating event such as binding to a negatively charged surface, the membrane localization of the extracellular serine proteases hepsin, matriptase, and prostasin provides them with a mechanism of concentrating, especially in special lipid domains such as that described below for prostasin. When not required to take action, the blood coagulation cascade serine protease zymogens and their eventual substrate for the ultimate functional output, fibrinogen, would coexist uneventfully in the same soluble environment.

The regulation of enzymatic activities and actions of the membrane-bound serine proteases will then likely involve the dynamically changing membrane structures during cellular functions and responses to the changes of the cell's environment, as well as the dynamic changes of the distribution of these proteases across the different domains in the cell's membranous continuum. In a fashion similar to the initiation of blood coagulation with the surface binding and concentrating of Factor XII, a plasma membrane localized proteolytic activation cascade involving at least a Type II transmembrane serine protease, matriptase, and a GPI-anchored extracellular serine protease, prostasin has recently been recognized. This membrane-localized extracellular serine protease proteolytic activation and action cascade will be discussed in further detail in the ensuing chapters.

Glycosylated-phosphatidylinositols (GPIs) are ubiquitous complex lipids discovered more than 30 years ago[11] and are found in all eukaryotic organisms. GPIs serve to anchor proteins in the membrane by the carboxyl-terminus following a post-translation modification. GPIs are synthesized in the lumen of the endoplasmic reticulum (ER), then anchored on the luminal surface of the ER. Addition of the GPI anchor to a protein takes place in the ER lumen via transamination. GPI-anchored proteins have a GPI-attachment site — the ω-site and a stretch of hydrophobic amino acid residues at the carboxyl terminus of the protein, known as the GPI anchor signal. The GPI transamidase binds to the hydrophobic signal peptide, cleaves off the GPI anchor signal segment and concomitantly replaces it with a GPI moiety. The attachment site varies in different GPI-anchored proteins (GPI-APs), but usually resides in a segment that has three consecutive amino acid residues with short side chains, followed by a short spacer sequence, then a carboxyl-terminal hydrophobic signal sequence. The hydrophobicity of the GPI anchor signal segment is less than those in the transmembrane domain of a Type II transmembrane protein but more than those in the secreted proteins with hydrophobic amino acid residues[12].

The GPI modification allows proteins to be anchored to the plasma membrane without the polypeptide passing through the membrane. The carboxyl terminus of the protein is covalently linked to the phosphatidylinositol in the outer leaflet of the plasma membrane via a phosphoethanolamine unit (Figure 2-2). Incorporation of [³H]-ethanolamine during GPI-protein synthesis is often used as a method to identify and ascertain proteins with a GPI anchor.

With a GPI anchorage, a protein performs functions on the external surface of the plasma membrane with better rotational freedom than the Type I and Type II transmembrane proteins. There are about 150 GPI-proteins in humans[13,14]. The GPI-APs participate in

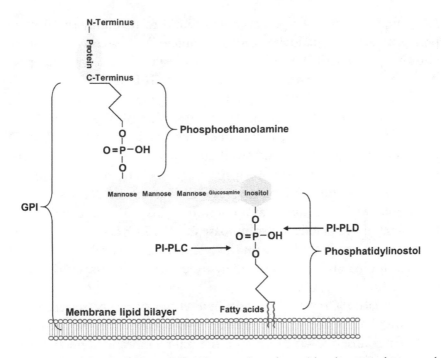

Figure 2-2. The GPI-APs consist of a protein polypeptide, the core glycan, and lipids.

many normal physiological processes, such as fertility, embryogenesis, morphogenesis, neurogenesis, and immunity, performing different and important functions including cell adhesion, receptor signal transduction, enzyme proteolysis, metabolism, and immune responses[15,16].

GPI-proteins are mostly clustered in specific domains of the plasma membrane, i.e., sphingolipid- and sterol-enriched membrane microdomains or rafts, and form homodimers[17,18]. This spatio-temporal organization allows them to interact with molecules in the vicinity, as well as molecules at a distance after GPI-specific phospholipase-mediated shedding. GPI-APs can be released from the cell surface by GPI-specific hydrolytic enzymes (GPIases), which have specificity towards their GPI-APs substrates. For example, the GPI-anchored urokinase plasminogen activator receptor (uPAR) can be shed by the glycerophosphodiesterase 3 (GDE3), a GPI-specific phospholipase

C[19]. The GPI-anchored prostasin was found to be highly sensitive to post-glycosylphosphatidylinositol attachment to proteins 6 (PGAP6, also known as TMEM8A) in an *in vitro* study. PGAP6 is a phospholipase A2 with a narrow substrate specificity to the GPI-APs[20,21].

In addition, both uPAR and prostasin can also be released from the cell membrane by the GPI-specific phospholipase D (GPI-PLD)[22,23]. Interestingly, it has been reported that the GPI-PLD prefers cleaving GPI-APs intracellularly within the secretory pathway but requires a detergent for the *in vitro* cleavage of cell surface GPI-APs[24,25], suggesting that the GPI-PLD does not cleave GPI-APs associated with the membrane microdomains. On the other hand, the bacterial PI-specific phospholipase C (PI-PLC) is the first enzyme identified to cleave GPI-APs on the cell surface[26] and release them off the membrane and has been widely used in *in vitro* assays to obtain GPI-anchor-free proteins.

Alternatively, the GPI-protein-lipid complex can be released into the extracellular space in the membrane-anchored form in the exosomes, and then re-inserted via fusion into the cell membrane of neighboring cells or other cells at a distant location[27]. With such mechanisms, they participate in functions of cell adhesion and cell-cell communication. Like most GPI-anchored proteins, prostasin can be released from the cell surface into the extracellular space in the form of exosome and the enzyme activity is preserved[28]. Exosomes are small membrane vesicles (30–150 nm in diameter) produced and released by most eukaryotic cells[29,30]. They contain specific sets of membranous and cellular proteins and nucleic acids depending on the cellular origin. Exosomes are capable of merging with other cells via specific receptor-ligand binding and membrane fusion or endocytosis. Thus, the exosomes can be viewed as special acellular envoys of the cell of origin to impose the properties and functions onto the recipient cells, a long-distance and remote mode of cell-cell communication. Exosomes are highly stable in the circulation and have low toxicity and low immunogenicity and have been investigated as tools in disease diagnosis (biomarkers), cargo delivery, and therapy[31].

References

1. Lewes GH (1860). In *The Physiology of Common Life (Volume II)*, William Blackwood and Sons, Edinburgh and London, 426–427.
2. Foy TM, Laman JD, Ledbetter JA, Aruffo A, Claassen E, Noelle RJ (1994). gp39-CD40 interactions are essential for germinal center formation and the development of B cell memory. *J Exp Med*. 180(1): 157–163.
3. Abercombie M, Heaysman J (1953). Observations on the social behaviour of cells in tissue culture: I. Speed of movement of chick heart fibroblasts in relation to their mutual contacts. *Cell*. 5(1):111–131.
4. Caughey GH, Raymond WW, Blount JL, Hau LW, Pallaoro M, Wolters PJ, Verghese GM (2000). Characterization of human gamma-tryptases, novel members of the chromosome 16p mast cell tryptase and prostasin gene families. *J Immunol*. 164(12):6566–6575.
5. Leytus SP, Loeb KR, Hagen FS, Kurachi K, Davie EW (1988). A novel trypsin-like serine protease (hepsin) with a putative transmembrane domain expressed by human liver and hepatoma cells. *Biochemistry*. 27(3):1067–1074.
6. Lin CY, Anders J, Johnson M, Sang QA, Dickson RB (1999). Molecular cloning of cDNA for matriptase, a matrix-degrading serine protease with trypsin-like activity. *J Biol Chem*. 274(26):18231–18236.
7. Lin CY, Anders J, Johnson M, Dickson RB (1999). Purification and characterization of a complex containing matriptase and a Kunitz-type serine protease inhibitor from human milk. *J Biol Chem*. 274(26):18237–18242.
8. Takeuchi T, Shuman MA, Craik CS (1999). Reverse biochemistry: Use of macromolecular protease inhibitors to dissect complex biological processes and identify a membrane-type serine protease in epithelial cancer and normal tissue. *Proc Natl Acad Sci USA*. 96(20):11054–11061.
9. Yu JX, Chao L, Chao J (1995). Molecular cloning, tissue-specific expression, and cellular localization of human prostasin mRNA. *J Biol Chem*. 270(22):13483–13489.
10. Chen LM, Skinner ML, Kauffman SW, Chao J, Chao L, Thaler CD, Chai KX (2001). Prostasin is a glycosylphosphatidylinositol-anchored active serine protease. *J Biol Chem*. 276(24):21434–21442.

11. Low MG, Saltiel AR (1988). Structural and functional roles of glyco-syl-phosphatidylinositol in membranes. *Science.* 239(4837):268–275.
12. Galian C, Björkholm P, Bulleid N, von Heijne G (2012). Efficient gly-cosylphosphatidylinositol (gpi) modification of membrane proteins requires a c-terminal anchoring signal of marginal hydrophobicity. *J Biol Chem.* 287(20):16399–16409.
13. UniProt Consortium (2015). UniProt: A hub for protein information. *Nucleic Acids Res.* 43(Database issue):D204–D212.
14. Kinoshita T (2020). Biosynthesis and biology of mammalian GPI-anchored proteins. *Open Biol.* 10(3):190290.
15. Fujihara Y, Ikawa M (2016). GPI-AP release in cellular, developmental, and reproductive biology. *J Lipid Res.* 57(4):538–545.
16. Heider S, Dangerfield JA, Metzner C (2016). Biomedical applica-tions of glycosylphosphatidylinositol-anchored proteins. *J Lipid Res.* 57(10):1778–1788.
17. Caiolfa VR, Zamai M, Malengo G, Andolfo A, Madsen CD, Sutin J, Digman MA, Gratton E, Blasi F, Sidenius N (2007). Monomer dimer dynamics and distribution of GPI-anchored uPAR are determined by cell surface protein assemblies. *J Cell Biol.* 179(5):1067–1082.
18. Suzuki KG, Kasai RS, Hirosawa KM, Nemoto YL, Ishibashi M, Miwa Y, Fujiwara TK, Kusumi A (2012). Transient GPI-anchored protein homodimers are units for raft organization and function. *Nat Chem Biol.* 8(9):774–783.
19. van Veen M, Matas-Rico E, van de Wetering K, Leyton-Puig D, Kedziora KM, De Lorenzi V, Stijf-Bultsma Y, van den Broek B, Jalink K, Sidenius N, Perrakis A, Moolenaar WH (2017). Negative regulation of urokinase receptor activity by a GPI-specific phospholipase C in breast cancer cells. *Elife.* 6:e23649.
20. Lee GH, Fujita M, Takaoka K, Murakami Y, Fujihara Y, Kanzawa N, Murakami KI, Kajikawa E, Takada Y, Saito K, Ikawa M, Hamada H, Maeda Y, Kinoshita T (2016). A GPI processing phospholipase A2, PGAP6, modulates Nodal signaling in embryos by shedding CRIPTO. *J Cell Biol.* 215(5):705–718.
21. Lee GH, Fujita M, Nakanishi H, Miyata H, Ikawa M, Maeda Y, Murakami Y, Kinoshita T (2020). PGAP6, a GPI-specific phospholipase A2, has narrow substrate specificity against GPI-anchored proteins. *J Biol Chem.* 295(42):14501–14509.
22. Wilhelm OG, Wilhelm S, Escott GM, Lutz V, Magdolen V, Schmitt M, Rifkin DB, Wilson EL, Graeff H, Brunner G (1999). Cellular glycosyl-

phosphatidylinositol-specific phospholipase D regulates urokinase receptor shedding and cell surface expression. *J Cell Physiol.* 180(2):225–235.

23. Verghese GM, Gutknecht MF, Caughey GH (2006). Prostasin regulates epithelial monolayer function: Cell-specific Gpld1-mediated secretion and functional role for GPI anchor. *Am J Physiol Cell Physiol.* 291(6):C1258–C1270.

24. Tsujioka H, Misumi Y, Takami N, Ikehara Y (1998). Posttranslational modification of glycosylphosphatidylinositol (GPI)-specific phospholipase D and its activity in cleavage of GPI anchors. *Biochem Biophys Res Commun.* 251:737–743.

25. Tsujioka H, Takami N, Misumi Y, Ikehara Y (1999). Intracellular cleavage of glycosylphosphatidylinositol by phospholipase D induces activation of protein kinase Calpha. *Biochem J.* 342:449–455.

26. Liu YS, Guo XY, Hirata T, Rong Y, Motooka D, Kitajima T, Murakami Y, Gao XD, Nakamura S, Kinoshita T, Fujita M (2018). N-Glycan–dependent protein folding and endoplasmic reticulum retention regulate GPI-anchor processing. *J Cell Biol.* 217(2):585–599.

27. Vidal M (2020). Exosomes and GPI-anchored proteins: Judicious pairs for investigating biomarkers from body fluids. *Adv Drug Delivery Rev.* 161–162:110–123.

28. Chen LM, Chai JC, Liu B, Strutt TM, McKinstry KK, Chai KX (2021). Prostasin regulates PD-L1 expression in human lung cancer cells. *Biosci Rep.* 41(7):BSR20211370.

29. Doyle LM, Wang MZ (2019). Overview of extracellular vesicles, their origin, composition, purpose, and methods for exosome isolation and analysis. *Cells.* 8:727.

30. Soekmadji C, Li B, Huang Y, Wang H, An T, Liu C, Pan W, Chen J, Cheung L, Falcon-Perez JM, Gho YS, Holthofer HB, Le MTN, Marcilla A, O'Driscoll L, Shekari F, Shen TL, Torrecilhas AC, Yan X, Yang F, Yin H, Xiao Y, Zhao Z, Zou X, Wang Q, Zheng L (2020). The future of extracellular vesicles as theranostics — an ISEV meeting report. *J Extracell Vesicles.* 9(1):1809766.

31. Dai J, Su Y, Zhong S, Cong L, Liu B, Yang J, Tao Y, He Z, Chen C, Jiang Y (2020). Exosomes: Key players in cancer and potential therapeutic strategy. *Signal Transduct Target Ther.* 5(1):145.

Chapter 3

Prostasin Serine Protease — 30 Years of Discoveries

3.1 How a new protein was identified and isolated

Human health and medicine have benefited enormously since the molecular revolution in the study of biology in the 1960s as a direct result of the determination of the structure of the genetic material, DNA, in the 1950s. A disease is clinically diagnosed, along with the identification of the system, organ, or tissue wherein a defect or malfunction is the potential cause. The defect is then reduced to a specific molecule, a protein, which is isolated for biochemical characterization. The molecular defect will be revealed and can guide our efforts at developing a remedy. At the clinical level, the observation is called a manifestation, but it is interchangeable with the genetics term "phenotype", which has two meanings: first, "pheno", which literally means "showing" and thus "can be observed" and second, "type", which means there are differences among individuals for a trait in a population. Typically, the easily accessible bodily fluids are the first to be investigated, and it is still true today in hospitals and clinics worldwide with blood, urine, and stool tests. An old but powerful example is the sickle cell disease, presented clinically as abnormal oxygen delivery from the circulatory system to tissues. The pathophysiological manifestation is the sickle-like shape of the patient's red blood cells. The biochemical cause is the clumping of the hemoglobin, which is the carrier of the blood oxygen. The red blood cells are anucleated but carry a large amount of hemoglobin, at >90% of the cell's dry weight. In an adult human, hemoglobin is composed of two α- and two β-globin subunits forming a tetramer quaternary structure, synthesized in the precursor cells, the reticulocytes.

The high globin content in the red blood cells facilitated their rather quick and easy isolation and purification to a high level of homogeneity, a prerequisite for biochemical characterization, including the determination of the amino acid sequence. The sequences of β-globin from sickle-cell patients and normal subjects were compared to show that the amino acid residue Glu in the 6th position of the polypeptide is replaced by a Val in the disease variant form. This change induces globin fiber clumping, which forces the cell shape to change, but more important, the clumping prevents access of oxygen. At this point, the picture of the disease manifestation and molecular mechanism can be described as complete, but it is not enough to bring benefits to the broader population and future generations. The knowledge of the genetic information at the DNA level is required to inform on the carriers and the risk of producing a child with sickle-cell. This became practical following the cloning of the human β-globin gene and the very first molecular diagnostic test was designed for the sickle-cell allele.

The discovery of the prostasin protein was not by design but rather serendipitous, just as the discovery of a family of serine proteases, known as the tissue kallikreins, in the early 1900s[1,2]. In 1925, a German surgeon Emil-Karl Frey injected human urine into dogs and observed a marked reduction in the arterial blood pressure. He reasoned that this blood pressure reduction was caused by a substance, F-substance, excreted in the kidney, likely a peptide hormone. The F-substance was initially named as "kallikrein" when the pancreas was speculated as its tissue origin[3,4]. The Greek word for pancreas is kallikreas. A decade later, kallikrein was identified as a proteolytic enzyme that releases the vasoactive peptide "DK" or kallidin (i.e., lys-bradykinin) from a plasma protein called kallidinogen or kininogen. The blood pressure lowering effect of human urine injected into dogs was mediated by lys-bradykinin and its further proteolytic derivatives via the engagement of bradykinin receptors on the blood vessel endothelial cells.

The "human urinary kallikrein", HUK, is now known as hK1 and its gene is designated as *KLK1* in the traditional human kallikrein gene family with three members, *KLK2* and *KLK3* being the other two. *KLK2* encodes human glandular kallikrein 1 (hGK-1), now known as hK2, and *KLK3* encodes the prostate-specific antigen (PSA), also known as hK3[5-8]. The new nomenclature was consolidated in the Kinin'91 meeting in 1991 in Munich, Germany[9]. At present, the number of genes in the tissue kallikrein gene family has increased from 3 to at least 15[10].

The discovery of prostasin was a serendipitous result of a research plan designed to isolate hGK-1. The gene and the cDNA of hGK-1 had been cloned and characterized, but the protein was never isolated[11-13]. Sequence analysis of the hGK-1 gene and cDNA indicated that the deduced hGK-1 protein should be very similar to the PSA. The hGK-1 mRNA was found, at that time with the available technology, to be expressed exclusively in the prostate gland[14].

The hGK-1 protein was predicated to be a serine protease, just like the PSA and tissue kallikrein in the same gene family. The three key amino acid residues in the charge-relay system required by serine proteases for the catalytic activity were conserved in the translated sequence of hGK-1 as well. Another assumption made was that the hGK-1 protein should be an acidic protein[15]. Therefore, the purification strategy was to aim for an acidic protein with trypsin-like activity in human seminal plasma which contains proteins secreted from the prostate. Acidic proteins carry negative charges on the protein surface in neutral or slightly alkaline solutions and bind to basic ion exchangers such as the diethylaminoethyl (DEAE)-Sepharose CL-6B resin, a matrix commonly used for protein purification by liquid chromatography. Aprotinin, also known as the bovine pancreatic trypsin inhibitor (BPTI), reversibly inhibits a trypsin-like protease's proteolytic activity. The aprotinin-coupled agarose resin is often used for isolating or removing trypsin-like proteins based on the affinity between the tryptic protease and aprotinin. This type of chromatography is called affinity chromatography and is the most efficient and effective in protein purification due to its simplicity and specificity to yield the final pure products.

In the first step, clarified seminal plasma was applied to the DEAE Sepharose CL-6B resin in a liquid chromatography column. Depending on the number of negative charges carried by a protein, the tightness of the binding between a protein and the DEAE matrix is different.

Proteins can be differentially eluted from the matrix by an increasing concentration gradient of salt (NaCl). The chloride ion displaces the bound proteins sequentially off the matrix by their affinities to the resin, from weak to strong. In the elution process, the presence of proteins was monitored with the absorption of ultraviolet light at 280 nm, recorded as a line graph showing peaks of high protein contents in the fractions of the eluted samples. To identify which fractions contain trypsin-like activities, samples were labeled with [^{14}C]diisopropyl fluorophosphates (DFP), a compound that binds to the active-site serine in serine proteases, or tested for trypsin-like activity using a synthetic tripeptidyl fluorogenic substrate D-Pro-Phe-Arg-MCA. Two peaks were identified to have trypsin-like activities in the eluted fractions, the peak eluted at NaCl concentrations between 0.15–0.25 M and the peak eluted at NaCl concentrations between 0.30–0.35 M. The fractions of the latter peak were confirmed to contain the human pancreatic/renal kallikrein 1 (hK1/HUK) protein.

The fractions from the first peak were combined and then further resolved by aprotinin-affinity chromatography to enrich and isolate the proteins with serine protease activity. The binding between a trypsin-like protease and aprotinin is rather tight and requires an acid solution with pH at ~2.5 to elute off the resin, followed by neutralization of the eluent. After these two steps, a protein with trypsin-like activity was purified to a high level of homogeneity[16].

3.2 Properties of the purified novel protein

Analysis of the purified protein by means of sodium dodecyl sulphate-polyacrylamide gel electrophoresis (SDS-PAGE) revealed a doublet of two closely migrating bands at ~40 kDa in its reduced form or at ~35 kDa in its non-reduced form. The two bands have an identical amino-terminal sequence, ITGGSSAVAGQWPWQVSITY, which did not match the sequence of any known proteins or translated gene products in the SwissPro or GenBank database, suggesting the discovery of a new protein. The new protein is acidic with isoelectric points (pI) ranging from 4.5–4.8, i.e., the protein carries no net electrical charge in this pH range. The extinction coefficient (E) of the protein is 1.63, as determined by measuring the absorbance at

Table 3-1. Properties of the new protein

Protein property		Synthetic Substrate	K_m (mM)	Inhibitor	IC_{50} (μM)
M.W.	~40 kDa reduced	D-Pro-Phe-Arg-MCA	108	Aprotinin	0.0018
	~35 kDa non-reduced	D-Val-Leu-Arg-MCA	255	Antipain	6.4
		D-Phe-Phe-Arg-MCA	827	Leupeptin	100
pI	4.5–4.8	Z-Gly-Pro-Arg-AFC	717	Benzamidine	860
E	1.63			SBTI	No inhibition

M.W.: molecular weight
pI: isoelectric point
E: extinction coefficient
K_m represents the substrate concentration at reaction of half V_{max}.
IC_{50} represents the inhibitor concentration at half prostasin activity inhibition.
SBTI: soybean trypsin inhibitor
V_{max}: maximal velocity
D-Pro-Phe-Arg-MCA was used in the inhibition assays.

205 nm and 280 nm[17]. The protein can be labeled with DFP, cleaves trypsin-like protease substrates, and is inhibited by a variety of serine protease inhibitors (summarized in Table 3-1).

In summary, the newly purified protein is an acidic, trypsin-like serine protease that was unknown before 1993. The purification method was simple and traditional, but the result was impactful. The key for this successful discovery was the source of the sample — human seminal plasma, which was later found to be the richest source of this protein in the human body (~8.61 μg/ml). Conversely, the unsuccessful attempt of isolating hGK-1 as initially planned may be attributed to the fact that in human seminal plasma, hGK-1 is usually in a complex form with inhibitors including protein C inhibitor (PCI), a serpin[18]. The hGK-1 protein in the complex form with its inhibitor loses its trypsin-like activity, unable to bind DFP and the surface charge of the protein complex could be much different, thus changing its binding to the DEAE matrix. In fact, the purification of hGK-1 was later made possible by applying human seminal plasma to CM Sepharose

CL-6B, a weak cation exchanger with the opposite mode of action to the weak anion exchanger DEAE Sepharose CL-6B and followed by an immune-affinity chromatography in which the matrix was coupled with an hGK-1-sepcific monoclonal antibody against a recombinant GST-fusion hGK-1 immunogen produced in bacteria[18,19].

3.3 Naming the newly discovered protein

The new protein was discovered and purified by Jack X. Yu, a graduate student in Dr. Julie Chao's laboratory in Medical University of South Carolina, USA[16]. Since the protein was isolated from the seminal plasma with a possible prostate origin, and has trypsin-like activity, the long name for the new protein is prostatic trypsin-like serine protease. The short-given name is prostasin. Prostasin purification in large quantities was made convenient by expressing a recombinant form in the HEK-293 cells using its full-length cDNA[20].

3.4 How the human prostasin cDNA and gene were cloned

The cDNA[21]

Once the new protein prostasin was purified to its homogeneity, it was fragmented by TPCK-trypsin digestion followed by fragment purification via reverse phase HPLC using a C18 column. A total of 15 fragments were obtained and five were subjected to amino-terminal sequence analysis. The amino acid sequences were used to design degenerate oligonucleotide primers. These primers were then used to generate a partial prostasin cDNA from a prostate cDNA library by means of the polymerase chain reaction (PCR). The amplified fragment, ~300 base pairs long, was sequenced with the dsDNA cycle sequencing system (Life Technologies, Inc.). New primers were designed according to the sequencing results and used in the determination of the full-length prostasin cDNA sequence by performing 3'-RACE (rapid amplification of cDNA ends) and 5'-RACE using human renal proximal tubular cell RNA as the template. The determined ends allowed the design of primers for cloning a full-length human prostasin cDNA by PCR, providing an essential tool for continued research in cell and animal models. The strategy of cloning the full-length prostasin cDNA is summarized in Figure 3-1. The structure of the cDNA and the predicted primary protein structure are shown as the colored boxes in Figure 3-1.

The gene[22]

For cloning the prostasin gene, two prostasin-specific primers in the coding region were used to amplify a 255-bp DNA fragment, which was used to screen a human genomic library in the Lamda Fix II vector (Stratagene Cloning Systems, La Jolla, CA). Two positive plaques were identified and confirmed from the 720,000 plaques screened. The two plaques were subjected to phage amplification and DNA purification, and the genomic DNA fragment from one of the two plaques were sequenced. The sequence in the flanking regions of the prostasin gene, 1.4 kilobases upstream and 1.2 kilobases downstream, was subsequently determined. The transcription initiation site was mapped by way of primer extension. A 9-kb genomic DNA fragment released from a prostasin gene clone in the Lambda phage vector was used to localize the prostasin gene to human chromosome 16p11.2 by fluorescence *in situ* hybridization (FISH) on metaphase chromosomes. The gene coding for prostasin is designated as *PRSS8*. The *PRSS8* gene structure and the chromosome location are illustrated in Figure 3-2.

The discovery of the prostasin protein and the cloning and localization of its gene onto a specific human chromosome[23] was an example of "forward genetics". The now somewhat out-of-fashion term "forward genetics" referred to the cloning of a protein-coding gene by starting at getting that protein, following a functional description, i.e., a phenotype. The ensuing characterization of the protein in the purified form would hopefully produce the amino acid sequence, or at least a part of that. The genetic information transfer from a protein-coding gene to its corresponding messenger RNA in the transcription step is precise and has a one-to-one residue-by-residue relationship. The genetic information transfer in the next step, translation, is also precise and obeys the universal genetic code with triplet-nucleotide codons. A few exceptions of the codons in the genetic code were uncovered in

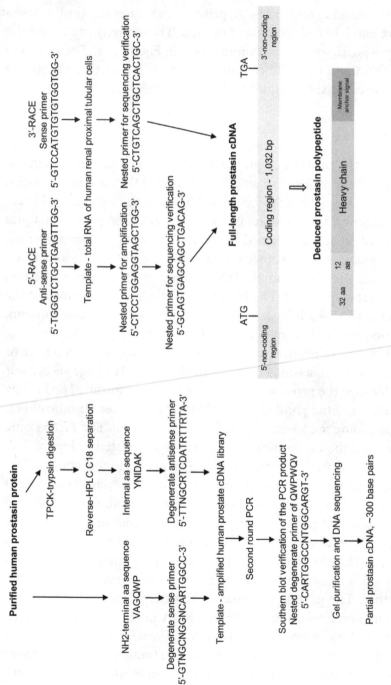

Figure 3-1. Strategy of cloning the full-length human prostasin cDNA and the deduced prostasin protein structure. The signal peptide is 32 aa (amino acid residues), the light chain is 12 aa, the putative membrane anchor is re-designated as a GPI anchor signal, which is replaced by a GPI anchor during the protein synthesis in the ER in epithelial cells.

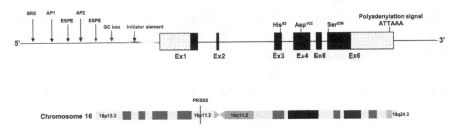

Figure 3-2. Prostasin gene structure and chromosome location.

the past year in bacteria. This "Central Dogma" of genetic information transfer is the foundation of molecular biology. In the reverse order, the information can be transferred from an RNA molecule to a DNA molecule, as in the case of the RNA genome in retroviruses, in a process called "reverse transcription" catalyzed by reverse transcriptases encoded in the viral genomes.

There is no natural process of information transfer, however, from the amino acid sequence of a protein to that of a nucleic acid, as noted by Francis Crick: "The central dogma of molecular biology deals with the detailed residue-by-residue transfer of sequential information. It states that such information cannot be transferred back from protein to either protein or nucleic acid". For nucleic acid transfer of genetic information, the precision in base pairing imposed by the active site of DNA or RNA polymerases is the mechanism for its high fidelity, whereas the reversibility of strand separation and re-association either *in vivo* or *in vitro* allows the access of the information-containing residues[24]. No such mechanism has been found for a potential protein to nucleic acid information transfer. In addition, proteins gain their biological function only after a precise three-dimensional structure is formed. This tertiary structure blocks off access of the information-containing residues, while unfolding of the structure is not reversible for all intents and purposes. As such, copying a protein molecule's residue-by-residue information would imply the destruction of that protein molecule.

So, for gene cloning by forward genetics to start with obtaining the protein in the pure form and then its amino acid sequence, what benefits does that amino acid sequence offer? A process known as "back translation" is the next step. Unlike reverse transcription, which is a naturally occurring process, back translation does not happen in nature but only on paper or in computers. The back-translated mRNA sequence, or by derivation, the coding sequence in the gene, is almost always "degenerate", i.e., having more than one possibility. This is caused by the degeneracy in the codons in the third or the wobble position, except for AUG/Met and UGG/Trp. For example, GGN, N = A, U, G, or C, codes for Gly, but for a Gly residue in the determined amino acid sequence of a protein (polypeptide), the codon could be any of the four, GGA, GGU, GGG, or GGC. The paper exercise of back translation cannot specify exactly which of the four is in the actual gene sequence coding for the Gly in that specific position in the protein (polypeptide).

Now expanding that to a string of amino acid residues in a peptide sequence, for example VAGQWP, an internal partial peptide sequence of prostasin, the possible codons for the six residues are 4 (Val), 4 (Ala), 4 (Gly), 2 (Gln), 1 (Trp), and 2 (Pro). Thus, a total of $4 \times 4 \times 4 \times 2 \times 1 \times 2 = 256$ different sequences are possible to be the actual corresponding sequence in the prostasin gene. The number 256 is referred to as the degree of degeneracy. The sense oligonucleotide primer used for amplification of the partial prostasin cDNA has the sequence of 5′-GTNGCNGGNCARTGGCC-3′ based on the internal amino acid sequence of prostasin VAGQWP. Even though the degeneracy of the primer is $4 \times 4 \times 4 \times 2 \times 1 \times 1$ (only the first two bases of the Pro codon were used) = 128, luckily, the most 3′-end of the primer has five unequivocal bases which greatly increased the priming efficiency of the primer to the template in the amplification reaction. The degeneracy of the antisense primer 5′-TTNGCRTCDATRTTRTA-3′ (corresponding to the internal amino acid sequence of YNIDAK) is 96.

Prostasin was abundant in the source material of seminal plasma, enabling its purification by a rather simple two-step procedure. Proteins that do not exist in large quantities or only exist in a transient manner will not allow this. The amino acid sequence obtained from tryptic fragments of the purified prostasin allowed deducement of candidate degenerate primer or probe sequences of relatively low degree of degeneracy, but not low enough to permit a cost-effective direct library screening.

Just prior to the identification of prostasin, the Chao laboratories at Medical University of South Carolina (MUSC) were successful with the molecular cloning of the serpin-class inhibitor of HUK, named kallistatin, by forward genetics. It began with the identification of a plasma protein capable of forming a covalent complex with a radiolabeled HUK, which became the functional assay to trace the candidate serpin for HUK in the purification steps. The amino acid sequence of fragments from the purified inhibitor permitted the design of degenerate synthetic oligonucleotides with relatively low degree of degeneracy, but also not low enough for a direct library screening. At the time, the groundbreaking molecular biological technique known as the "polymerase chain reaction" (PCR), invented by the late Kary Mullis, was making its way into molecular biology laboratories following the discovery and commercialization of the heat resistant Taq DNA polymerase. In an unprecedented attempt at that time, paired opposing degenerate oligos derived from different portions of the purified inhibitor were used in consecutive PCR with the phage DNA mixture from a cDNA library of the human HepG2 hepatoma cell line as the initial templates. These were the products of amplification by PCR using the vector primers. The products of each round of PCR were then used as the templates for the ensuing rounds until a dominant band was visualized in agarose gel electrophoresis, at the end of the fourth round. This amplified DNA fragment was then sequenced with a third degenerate oligo using the Sanger method. A specific DNA sequence was obtained, and its translated amino acid sequence matched that of the peptide fragments of the purified inhibitor. The confirmed sequence allowed the amplification and cloning of a partial cDNA of kallistatin, and the isolation of a full-length cDNA clone from the HepG2 library[25,26].

The best way to understand and appreciate "forward genetics" in the "directional sense" is that the journey goes forward to the destination of getting the genetic information. In contrast, the practice of "reverse genetics" starts with the genetic information, via a functional phenotypic association to genetic markers, sites in the genome showing variations among the population. It is often synonymous to "positional cloning" or "linkage analysis" but some variations on the theme were proven to be just as effective. Completely independent to the serendipitous discovery of prostasin from human seminal plasma and the cloning of its gene via forward genetics, prostasin, aka channel-activating protease 1 (CAP1), was cloned by a variation of reverse genetics several years later in 1997[27]. In pursuit of a candidate protease that activates the epithelial sodium channel (ENaC) in the same way as trypsin, a functional complementation assay measuring the ENaC activity was established with Xenopus oocytes. An A6 Xenopus kidney cell cDNA library was functionally screened by oocyte co-injection of cRNA transcribed *in vitro* from pools of the cDNA along with the cRNA for the αβγ subunits of the Xenopus ENaC. The cloned cDNA of CAP1, by comparison of sequence and the translated amino acid sequence was determined to be the orthologue of prostasin in the frog. Unlike the classical examples of positional cloning by reverse genetics, such as the Huntingtin and the CFTR (cystic fibrosis transmembrane conductance regulator) genes, in which the determination of the genomic region with a variant 100% associated with the disease phenotypes revealed no information on the structure of the candidate genes, the functional cloning of CAP1/prostasin helped establish a biological function of the genetic information contained in the cDNA clone with a translated putative protein sequence.

Genes that were cloned by way of forward genetics require a reverse genetics validation of its causal relationship to the initially described biological function. This can be achieved *in vitro* in tissue cultured cells or *in vivo* in animal models by either a gain of expression or a loss of expression via the modification of the gene or manipulation of gene expression. In addition to its ENaC activating function, many more putative functions in biology and pathobiology have been implicated for prostasin and these will be addressed in later chapters.

References

1. Frey EK (1926). Zusammenhänge zwischen Herzabeit und Nierentätigkeit. *Arch Klin Chir*. 142:663–669.
2. Frey EK, Kraut H (1928). Ein neues Kreislaufhormon und seine Wirkung. *Arch Exp Pathol Pharamakol*. 133:1–56.
3. Kraut H, Frey EK, Werle E (1930). Der Nachweis eines Kreislaufhormon in de Pankreasdruse. *Hoppe-Seyler's Z Physiol Chem*. 189:97–106.

4. Werle E (1934). Zur Kenntnis des haushalts des Kallikreins. *Biochem Z.* 269:415–434.
5. Riegman PHJ, Vlietstra RJ, Suurmeijer L, Cleutjens CBJM, Trapman J (1992). Characterization of the human kallikrein locus. *Genomics.* 14(1):6–11.
6. Chao J (2013). Chapter 607 — Human Kallikrein 1, Tissue Kallikrein. In *Handbook of Proteolytic Enzymes (Third Edition)*, Rawlings ND, Salvesen G (eds.), Academic Press, 2757–2761.
7. Chao J, Chen LM, Chai KX (2013). Chapter 608 — Human Kallikrein-related Peptidase 2. In *Handbook of Proteolytic Enzymes (Third Edition)*, Rawlings ND, Salvesen G (eds.), Academic Press, 2762–2765.
8. Chao J, Chai KX, Chen LM (2013). Chapter 609 — Human Kallikrein-related Peptidase 3, the Prostate-specific Antigen. In *Handbook of Proteolytic Enzymes (Third Edition)*, Rawlings ND, Salvesen G (eds.), Academic Press, 2765–2768.
9. Berg T, Bradshaw RA, Carretero OA, Chao J, Chao L, Clements JA, Fahnestock M, Fritz H, Gauthier F, MacDonald RJ, Margolius HS, Morris BJ, Richards RI, Scicli AG (1992). A common nomenclature for members of the tissue (glandular) kallikrein gene families. *Agents Actions Suppl.* 38(Pt 1):19–25.
10. Yousef GM, Diamandis EP (2001). The new human tissue kallikrein gene family: structure, function, and association to disease. *Endocr Rev.* 22(2):184–204.
11. Schedlich LJ, Bennetts BH, Morris BJ (1987). Primary structure of a human glandular kallikrein gene. *DNA.* 6(5):429–437.
12. Paradis G, Tremblay RR, Dubé JY (1989). Looking for human glandular kallikrein-1 in the prostate. *Prostate.* 15(4):343–353.
13. Young CY, Andrews PE, Montgomery BT, Tindall DJ (1992). Tissue-specific and hormonal regulation of human prostate-specific glandular kallikrein. *Biochemistry.* 31(3):818–824.
14. Morris BJ (1989). hGK-1: A kallikrein gene expressed in human prostate. *Clin Exp Pharmacol Physiol.* 16(4):345–351.
15. Moore BW (1969). Acidic Proteins. In *Chemical Architecture of the Nervous System*, Lajtha A (ed.), Springer, Boston, MA, 93–99.
16. Yu JX, Chao L, Chao J (1994). Prostasin is a novel human serine protease from seminal fluid. Purification, tissue distribution, and localization in prostate gland. *J Biol Chem.* 269(29):18843–18848.
17. ... JF, Duine JA (1985). Determination of absorption coefficient ... proteins by conventional ultraviolet spectrophotometry ... hy combined with multiwavelength detection. ...04.

18. Deperthes D, Chapdelaine P, Tremblay RR, Brunet C, Berton J, Hébert J, Lazure C, Dubé JY (1995). Isolation of prostatic kallikrein hK2, also known as hGK-1, in human seminal plasma. *Biochim Biophys Acta.* 1245(3):311–316.

19. Frenette G, Deperthes D, Tremblay RR, Lazure C, Dubé JY (1997). Purification of enzymatically active kallikrein hK2 from human seminal plasma. *Biochim Biophys Acta.* 1334(1):109–115.

20. Chen LM, Skinner ML, Kauffman SW, Chao J, Chao L, Thaler CD, Chai KX (2001). Prostasin is a glycosylphosphatidylinositol-anchored active serine protease. *J Biol Chem.* 276(24):21434–21442.

21. Yu JX, Chao L, Chao J (1995). Molecular cloning, tissue-specific expression, and cellular localization of human prostasin mRNA. *J Biol Chem.* 270(22):13483–13489.

22. Yu JX, Chao L, Ward DC, Chao J (1996). Structure and chromosomal localization of the human prostasin (PRSS8) gene. *Genomics.* 32(3):334–340.

23. Chao J, Chen LM, Chai KX (2013). Chapter 658 — Prostasin. In *Handbook of Proteolytic Enzymes (Third Edition)*, Rawlings ND, Salvesen G (eds.), Academic Press, 3011–3014.

24. Britten RJ, Kohne DE (1968). Repeated sequences in DNA. Hundreds of thousands of copies of DNA sequences have been incorporated into the genomes of higher organisms. *Science.* 161(3841):529–540.

25. Zhou GX, Chao L, Chao J (1992). Kallistatin: A novel human tissue kallikrein inhibitor. Purification, characterization, and reactive center sequence. *J Biol Chem.* 267(36):25873–25880.

26. Chai KX, Chen LM, Chao J, Chao L (1993). Kallistatin: A novel human serine proteinase inhibitor. Molecular cloning, tissue distribution, and expression in Escherichia coli. *J Biol Chem.* 268(32):24498–24505.

27. Vallet V, Chraibi A, Gaeggeler HP, Horisberger JD, Rossier BC (1997). An epithelial serine protease activates the amiloride-sensitive sodium channel. *Nature.* 389(6651):607–610.

Chapter 4

The Basic Molecular Information
on Prostasin

The basic molecular information on the prostasin serine protease, along the axis of genetic information transfer in the Central Dogma, is provided here for both the human and the mouse homologues. While the information on the human form is essential for understanding the expression and functions of prostasin for health and medicine, that on the mouse is also critical because a good amount of our understanding came from studying the mouse form in the animal models.

4.1 The prostasin gene in the human and the mouse

The human prostasin gene[1] is formally listed as Human Gene *PRSS8* (ENSG00000052344.16; GENCODE V39), with the genomic position defined by: hg38 chr16:31,131,433-31,135,727 encoding a 4,295-nt transcript (ENST00000317508.11) which includes the untranslated regions (UTRs). The coding region of the *PRSS8* gene is defined by: hg38 chr16:31,132,009-31,135,498 at 3,490 nucleotides.

The *PRSS8* gene is single-copied and localized on chromosome 16 in band p11.2 (16p11.2), close to the center. Human chromosome 16 spans more than 90 million base pairs containing 800–900 genes for making proteins and represents ~3% of the total genomic DNA. Interestingly, chromosome 16 has one of the highest levels of segmentally duplicated sequence among the human autosomes, especially at the 16p11 pericentromeric region[2]. Conversely, deletion of DNA in the 16p11 region has also been documented[3].

The 16p11.2 deletion syndrome[3]

The 16p11.2 deletion associated disease syndrome is a disorder of delayed development in the neural system resulting in intellectual disabilities, such as impaired communication, socialization, speech, and language expressive skills, as well as autistic behaviors. The microdeletions observed in patients with the 16p11.2 deletion syndrome are within ~600 kilobases (kb) of DNA, covering 29 known genes, including the *PRSS8* gene. Different patients display microdeletions of different genes. For autistic traits, the deletion of a small segment with five genes is sufficient. Some individuals may have a microdeletion without manifesting any associated health or behavioral problems. Therefore, the prevalence of this syndrome may be underestimated, but nevertheless, is ~3 in 10,000. Most of the manifested cases are not inherited, indicating a mechanism of deletion during gametogenesis or early embryonic development. The deletion of one copy of chromosome 16 is sufficient to cause the syndrome, indicating haploinsufficiency for the deleted genes.

The 16p11.2 duplication[4]

The 600-kb DNA segment may also display duplication in the same region. Interestingly, the symptoms associated with the duplications often mirror those with microdeletions in the same 600-kb DNA segment, but the symptoms are usually milder in the affected individuals with duplications. Again, not all subjects with duplications will necessarily manifest physical or behavioral abnormalities. To date there has been no study that directly points to a causative role for the *PRSS8* gene in either the deletion or the duplication cases involving the 600-kb 16p11.2 region.

No major deletions or chromosomal abnormalities have been reported for the human prostasin gene. Knocking out both copies of the prostasin gene is embryonically lethal in mouse models. Knocking out a single copy does not affect the heterozygotes, therefore, the prostasin gene is haplosufficient[5]. A single case of a fusion gene, *PRSS8-S100A14* (FusionGDB2 ID:29018) was reported between *PRSS8* and *S100A14*, encoding the S100 calcium binding protein A14. A search with the gene symbol *PRSS8* in the most recent Build 155 of the NCBI Short Genetic Variation Database dbSNP (June 16, 2021) retrieves 2,593 entries from the total of >3.34 billion variations, with the great majority being single-nucleotide polymorphisms (SNPs) along with some small insertions and deletions (indel's). Remarkably, none of the variations is currently indexed as being associated with a phenotype in the Online Mendelian Inheritance in Man (OMIM), a compendium of human genes and genetic phenotypes for all known Mendelian disorders and over 12,000 genes.

This lack of clinical phenotype association may indicate the essential functional role of prostasin throughout the personal development from the early embryonic stages, but may also be a reflection of the status that the genetic association with the *PRSS8* variants has not been adequately studied. Several genome-wide association studies (GWAS) suggested an association of variants in the *KAT8* region of human chromosome 16 with Alzheimer disease. In 2021, Pietzner and colleagues performed a genome-proteome-wide association study and identified variants strongly associated with Alzheimer's disease in the prostasin gene in the *KAT8* region[6]. The *KAT8* gene (chr16:31,115,754-31,131,393), encoding lysine histone acetyltransferase 8, is immediately adjacent in a tail-to-tail fashion to the prostasin gene (chr16:31,131,433-31,135,727) in chromosome 16p11.2, making it very challenging to assign a true genetic variant-to-phenotype relationship as any genomic perturbation herein may impact both genes in their expression.

The genes encoding the homologues of prostasin are highly conserved with the closest relative being the rhesus monkey prostasin gene, presenting a high degree of sequence identity across the entire gene. The mouse, dog, and elephant prostasin genes are also highly homologous to the human counterpart, with the sequence identities concentrated in the coding region. The prostasin gene of the chicken would have a much-reduced sequence identity shared with the human counterpart. The mouse prostasin gene[7,8] *Prss8* is located on chromosome 7 at chr7:127,524,888-127,529,276 bp (the minus-strand, in the Ensembl annotation of GRCm39) at 4,389 nt/bp in length, while the coding region is defined by chr7:127,525,498-127,529,054 at 3,557 nt/bp. It also has a 6-exon gene organization and its 5'- and 3'-UTRs are similar in lengths to those in the human *PRSS8* gene. A variant form of the *Prss8* gene has a 7-exon organization, with the first exon split into two portions. The human disease autosomal recessive congenital ichthyosis is modeled in the mouse with mutations artificially created in the *Prss8* gene[9]. A total of 18 mutations in the *Prss8* gene have been studied with various phenotypic outcomes.

The originally cloned *PRSS8* gene fragment[10] is 7 kilobases (kb) long consisting of a 1.4-kb 5'-flanking region, a 4.4-kb *PRSS8* structural gene with 6 exons interrupted by 5 introns, and a 1.2-kb 3'-flanking region. There is no TATA-box identified in the 5'-flanking region of the prostasin gene, but there is an initiator element which presumably starts the transcription. The initiator element is similar to that identified in the murine terminal deoxynucleotidyl transferase gene. Several transcription regulatory elements are identified in the 5'-flanking region of the gene (Figure 3-2). These elements serve as regulator protein binding sites to enhance or repress the prostasin gene expression. The AP2 site, responsive to regulation by phorbol esters such as phorbol 13-acetate 12-myristate (PMA) and by protein kinase C (PKC), is upstream of the transcription initiator element. Two erythroid-specific promoter elements (ESPE) flank the AP2 site. A sterol regulatory element (SRE) is the most upstream element identified. The SRE is a binding site for mature sterol-regulatory element-binding proteins (SREBPs). A variant GC box and a variant AP1 site are present in the 5'-flanking region upstream from the transcription initiator element. A highly AC-rich region spanning more than 300 base pairs (bp) is located just upstream from the transcription initiator element.

New SRE sites and CpG dinucleotide-enriched regions were identified in the ensuing years[11-13], which are the molecular basis for prostasin expression regulation. The human prostasin gene is transcriptionally regulated by promoter DNA methylation and associated histone modifications, the transcription repressors Slug and Snail, sterol-regulatory element-binding protein-2 (SREBP-2) and transforming growth factor beta 1 (TGFβ1)[14-16]. The long non-coding RNAs (lncRNAs) may be a regulating mechanism as well[17-19]. The detailed molecular mechanisms mediating the expression regulation of the *PRSS8* gene in different tissue and cellular contexts will be addressed in later chapters.

4.2 The mRNA transcript

The human prostasin mRNA (PRSS8) is listed as RefSeq NM_002773. The originally cloned human prostasin cDNA[20] was a 1,742-bp DNA fragment consisting of a 138-bp 5'-untranslated region (UTR), a 1,032-bp open-reading frame from the six exons, and a 572-bp 3'-UTR. The transcription initiation site of the *PRSS8* gene is 332-nt upstream from the translational start codon AUG. The three key amino acid residues constituting the catalytic triad (aka, the charge relay system) required for prostasin's catalytic activity are encoded in exons III (His85), IV (Asp134), and VI (Ser238) in the corresponding coding region of the *PRSS8* gene. By means of reverse transcription coupled with Southern blotting using specific oligonucleotides, the human prostasin transcript was detected from the total cellular RNA extracted from the prostate, liver, salivary glands, kidney, lung, pancreas, and colon, but was not detected from the RNA of the testis, ovary, spleen, uterus, brain cortex, muscle, heart atrium and ventricle, aorta, vein, or artery. The prostasin transcript was also detected from the total cellular RNA of several human cell lines, including those of lung bronchi, renal proximal tubules, prostate cancer (LNCaP), but was not detected in human blood cells such as the lymphocytes or polymorphonuclear leukocytes (PMNs). The sources of RNA in the initial screening of prostasin transcript expression were based on the immediate availability.

With the modern technique of RNA-Seq, a next-generation (next-gen) sequencing (NGS) technique that determines the types and copy numbers of RNA transcripts more accurately and completely, additional human tissue sites such as the breast, bladder, cervix, esophagus (mucosa), skin, small intestine (terminal ileum), stomach, thyroid, and vagina were reported to express the prostasin transcript. The data were part of The Genotype-Tissue Expression (GTEx) project. The colon was shown to express the highest median amount among the 57 tissues tested. The localization of the prostasin mRNA is almost exclusively in the epithelial cells of the prostate, kidney, lung, and colon. Expression of prostasin has been identified in the epithelial cells in the ovary and uterus (endometrium).

The mouse prostasin mRNA (Prss8) is listed as RefSeq NM_133351. The mouse prostasin mRNA transcript has been investigated in a broader range of tissues and cell types owing to the availability of the experimental material, at 132 in total, as described at the Mouse Genome Informatics website[9].

The untranslated regions of the human prostasin mRNA are predicted to form highly compact secondary stem-loop structures, with fold energy at −77.00 and −227.80 kcal/mole for those in the 5'- and the 3'-UTR, respectively, using the RNAfold program of the Vienna RNA Packages. The implications of the high energy, i.e., complex and stable secondary structures in the UTRs will be in the half-life and the accessibility to the translational machinery. Currently, there is very limited information from research on the impact of the prostasin UTRs to its expression, with one report on Argonaut 2 (AGO2) binding in the 3'-UTR not affecting the mRNA expression in cells with AGO2 knockout. For the mouse prostasin 5'- and 3'-UTRs, the secondary structure fold energy is −68.00 kcal/mole and −193.70 kcal/mole, respectively.

With the completion and refinement of the genomes of many mammalian species, it is now clear that the mammalian genomes contain overlapping genes, which were thought to be seen only in the genomes of prokaryotes. In the *PRSS8* position hg38 chr16:31,131,433-31,135,727, a novel transcript of ENST00000563605.1 was described between 31,131,432 and 31,131,877 and is given a Human Gene Code ENSG00000261385. This transcript is a lncRNA antisense to the 3'-UTR of the proper PRSS8 transcript. This lncRNA is apparently expressed in a coordinated manner in the tissues and cells where the proper PRSS8 transcript is found. It is not clear at the present time if this lncRNA may affect the translation of the proper PRSS8 mRNA or its stability.

In the mouse, a functional protein-coding gene overlaps with the *Prss8* gene in the genomic position. The *Kat8* gene is located at position chr7:127,511,688-127,525,009 with a length of 13,322 nt/bp. *Kat8* encodes K (lysine) acetyltransferase 8, with its mRNA listed as RefSeq NM_026370. *Kat8* overlaps on the plus strand with Exon 6 of the *Prss8* gene in the 3'-UTR on the minus strand. This overlapping gene structure for *Kat8* and *Prss8* in the mouse genome is conserved in the rat genome, as well. The Kat8 histone acetyltransferase is essential for mouse oocyte development, functioning as a regulator of the reactive oxygen species levels. It is also expressed at a high level during sperm development. The overlap of the *Prss8* and *Kat8* genes in the mouse genome must be carefully contemplated upon in any efforts of gene knockout (KO) of *Prss8* to study its biological effects. It may not be adequate to just avoid removing any of the nucleotides in the defined *Kat8* gene region. The *Prss8* gene is in the immediate downstream of the *Kat8* and a perturbation to the genomic sequence and therefore, the chromatin structure may affect the expression of the *Kat8* gene after all. The minimum amount of caution in such experiments would be to at least monitor the *Kat8* gene expression changes in animals with a *Prss8* KO.

4.3 The protein[21]

Analysis of the amino acid sequence deduced from the prostasin cDNA sequence with the aid of the Kyte & Doolittle hydropathy index[22] revealed two hydrophobic regions in the prostasin protein. The amino-terminal hydrophobic region represents the signal peptide for processing the pre-pro-prostasin to the pro-prostasin, as seen for other serine proteases[23]. The presence of a carboxyl-terminal hydrophobic region suggests that prostasin may be membrane-anchored to the plasma membrane at the carboxyl terminus. Subsequently, prostasin was proven to be attached to the cell surface membrane via a glycosylphosphatidylinositol (GPI) anchor[24]. The GPI moiety uses ethanolamine as a linker between the carboxyl-terminal amino acid residue and the glycan structure during the synthesis of GPI-anchored proteins. This structural characteristic is used experimentally to show the GPI-anchorage of an extracellular protein. The tritium-labeled [^{3}H]-ethanolamine was used in the synthesis of a recombinant human prostasin protein (r-prostasin) in the human embryonic kidney

293 (HEK-293) cells stably harboring an episomal plasmid carrying the human prostasin cDNA. The r-prostasin was shown to be labeled at the ethanolamine in the GPI with [1-³H]-ethan-1-ol-2-amine hydrochloride. Subcellular fractionation and GPI releasing assays confirmed that prostasin is a GPI-anchored protein, not a transmembrane protein or linked to another membrane-bound protein.

Prostasin is synthesized as a pre-pro-enzyme of 343 amino acid residues. The 32-residue signal peptide is removed upon cleavage, generating the pro-prostasin, which is then processed by a specific cleavage between Arg12 (R44 when including the signal peptide) and Ile13 to produce a mature prostasin with two chains — a light chain and a heavy chain held together by a disulfide bond. Prostasin has one potential N-linked glycosylation site at Asn127. The three-dimensional (3-D) structure of the human prostasin predicted by ModBase[25] shows compact views of β-sheets and a hollow top view with two α-helices on the exterior of the modeled structure.

Prostasin is active as a serine protease in its membrane-anchored form and when released apically to the environment in the exosome form[26]. The prostasin serine protease can be shed off from the membrane without the GPI moiety via unknown mechanisms. The cleavage that releases the free prostasin is between Arg290 and Pro291, based on the carboxyl-terminal amino acid sequence analysis using carboxypeptidases on the free prostasin purified from human seminal plasma[21].

The active prostasin protein is very sensitive to the reversible serine protease inhibitor aprotinin (IC50: 1.8×10^{-9}M), but not very much to the soybean trypsin inhibitor (SBTI). This characteristic can be used to distinguish prostasin from other serine proteases that are sensitive to the SBTI, e.g., plasma kallikrein[27,28].

The prostasin protein is found at high levels in the prostate gland and the seminal plasma (~8.6 μg/ml), at a moderate level in the urine (~0.2 μg/ml), and at much lower levels in other tissues such as the colon, lung, kidney, pancreas, salivary gland, liver, and bronchi. The prostasin protein is mainly localized in the polarized epithelial cells towards the lumen of glandular tissues with polarized cells, as shown by immunohistochemistry from various studies[21,29].

A recombinant human prostasin (r-prostasin) in the purified and active soluble form was obtained by maintaining the human prostasin cDNA in the pREP8 expression vector (Invitrogen®) in the HEK-293/EBNA cell line in the episomal setting[24]. This unique class of plasmid vectors contain the Epstein-Barr virus replication origin (oriP) and its nuclear antigen EBNA-1 gene to enable episomal replication in mammalian cell lines. The full-length cDNA containing 209 base pairs of the 5'-UTR, 1,032 base pairs of the coding region, and 655 base pairs of the 3'-UTR, was amplified from the RNA of the LNCaP human prostate cancer cell line by means of reverse-transcription and polymerase chain reaction (RT-PCR). The expression of the human prostasin cDNA is under the control of the Rous Sarcoma Virus long terminal repeat (RSV-LTR) enhancer/promoter and is maintained episomally in the HEK-293/EBNA cells under L-histidinol dihydrochloride selection. Expression and purification of the active prostasin serine protease domain using a baculovirus system was reported by Shipway and colleagues in 2004[30]. Rickert and colleagues crystalized recombinant human prostasin heavy chain purified from *E. coli* cells in 2008[31], while Spraggon and colleagues in 2009 produced and purified one from the SF9 insect cells[32]. The availability of this free and soluble form of the active prostasin serine protease is very important in determining the substrate cleavage site amino acid residue specificity using synthetic or natural substrates. It is also important to point out that the results obtained from studying this form of the prostasin enzyme may not be directly transferable to the membrane-anchored form, where the potential differences in its conformation and the membrane topology must be taken into consideration.

References

1. UCSC Genome Browser on Human (GRCh38/hg38). https:// genome.ucsc.edu/cgi-bin/hgTracks?db=hg38&lastVirtModeType=default&lastVirtModeExtraState=&virtModeType=default&virtMode=0&nonVirtPosition=&position=chr16%3A31131433%2D31-135727&hgsid=1288578493_vFmoHm10RsNKrWS67NCGuKvAnrub
2. Martin J, Han C, Gordon LA, Terry A, Prabhakar S, She X, Xie G, Hellsten U, Chan YM, Altherr M, Couronne O, Aerts A, Bajorek E, Black S, Blumer H, Branscomb E, Brown NC, Bruno WJ, Buckingham JM,

Callen DF, Campbell CS, Campbell ML, Campbell EW, Caoile C, Challacombe JF, Chasteen LA, Chertkov O, Chi HC, Christensen M, Clark LM, Cohn JD, Denys M, Detter JC, Dickson M, Dimitrijevic-Bussod M, Escobar J, Fawcett JJ, Flowers D, Fotopulos D, Glavina T, Gomez M, Gonzales E, Goodstein D, Goodwin LA, Grady DL, Grigoriev I, Groza M, Hammon N, Hawkins T, Haydu L, Hildebrand CE, Huang W, Israni S, Jett J, Jewett PB, Kadner K, Kimball H, Kobayashi A, Krawczyk MC, Leyba T, Longmire JL, Lopez F, Lou Y, Lowry S, Ludeman T, Manohar CF, Mark GA, McMurray KL, Meincke LJ, Morgan J, Moyzis RK, Mundt MO, Munk AC, Nandkeshwar RD, Pitluck S, Pollard M, Predki P, Parson-Quintana B, Ramirez L, Rash S, Retterer J, Ricke DO, Robinson DL, Rodriguez A, Salamov A, Saunders EH, Scott D, Shough T, Stallings RL, Stalvey M, Sutherland RD, Tapia R, Tesmer JG, Thayer N, Thompson LS, Tice H, Torney DC, Tran-Gyamfi M, Tsai M, Ulanovsky LE, Ustaszewska A, Vo N, White PS, Williams AL, Wills PL, Wu JR, Wu K, Yang J, Dejong P, Bruce D, Doggett NA, Deaven L, Schmutz J, Grimwood J, Richardson P, Rokhsar DS, Eichler EE, Gilna P, Lucas SM, Myers RM, Rubin EM, Pennacchio LA (2004). The sequence and analysis of duplication-rich human chromosome 16. *Nature*. 432(7020): 988–994.

3. Ballif BC, Hornor SA, Jenkins E, Madan-Khetarpal S, Surti U, Jackson KE, Asamoah A, Brock PL, Gowans GC, Conway RL, Graham JM Jr, Medne L, Zackai EH, Shaikh TH, Geoghegan J, Selzer RR, Eis PS, Bejjani BA, Shaffer LG (2007). Discovery of a previously unrecognized microdeletion syndrome of 16p11. *Nat Genet*. 39:1071–1073.

4. D'Angelo D, Lebon S, Chen Q, Martin-Brevet S, Snyder LG, Hippolyte L, Hanson E, Maillard AM, Faucett WA, Macé A, Pain A, Bernier R, Chawner SJ, David A, Andrieux J, Aylward E, Baujat G, Caldeira I, Conus P, Ferrari C, Forzano F, Gérard M, Goin-Kochel RP, Grant E, Hunter JV, Isidor B, Jacquette A, Jønch AE, Keren B, Lacombe D, Le Caignec C, Martin CL, Männik K, Metspalu A, Mignot C, Mukherjee P, Owen MJ, Passeggeri M, Rooryck-Thambo C, Rosenfeld JA, Spence SJ, Steinman KJ, Tjernagel J, Van Haelst M, Shen Y, Draganski B, Sherr EH, Ledbetter DH, van den Bree MB, Beckmann JS, Spiro JE, Reymond A, Jacquemont S, Chung WK, et al. (2016). Defining the effect of the 16p11.2 duplication on cognition, behavior, and medical comorbidities. *JAMA Psychiatry*. 73:20–30.

5. Hummler E, Dousse A, Rieder A, Stehle JC, Rubera I, Osterheld MC, Beermann F, Frateschi S, Charles RP, (2013). The channel-activating

protease CAP1/Prss8 is required for placental labyrinth maturation. *PLoS One.* 8(2):e55796.

6. Pietzner M, Wheeler E, Carrasco-Zanini J, Cortes A, Koprulu M, Wörheide MA, Oerton E, Cook J, Stewart ID, Kerrison ND, Luan J, Raffler J, Arnold M, Ailt W, O'Rahilly S, Kastenmüller G, Gamazon ER, Hingorani AD, Scott RA, Wareham NJ, Langenberg C (2021). Mapping the proteo-genomic convergence of human diseases. *Science.* 374(6569):eabj1541.

7. Verghese GM, Tong ZY, Bhagwandin V, Caughey GH (2004). Mouse prostasin gene structure, promoter analysis, and restricted expression in lung and kidney. *Am J Respir Cell Mol Biol.* 30(4):519–529.

8. UCSC Genome Browser on Mouse (GRCm39/mm39). https://genome.ucsc.edu/cgi-bin/hgTracks?db=mm39&lastVirtModeType=default&lastVirtModeExtraState=&virtModeType=default&virtMode=0&nonVirtPosition=&position=chr7%3A127524888%2D127529276&hgsid=1288707411_0KpXged7pPFAzRhcnoMb3ma6aXXo

9. http://www.informatics.jax.org/marker/MGI:1923810

10. Yu JX, Chao L, Ward DC, Chao J (1996). Structure and chromosomal localization of the human prostasin (PRSS8) gene. *Genomics.* 32(3):334–340.

11. Chen LM, Chai KX (2002). Prostasin serine protease inhibits breast cancer invasiveness and is transcriptionally regulated by promoter DNA methylation. *Int J Cancer.* 97(3):323–329.

12. Chen LM, Zhang X, Chai KX (2004). Regulation of prostasin expression and function in the prostate. *Prostate.* 59(1):1–12.

13. Chen M, Chen LM, Chai KX (2006). Mechanisms of sterol regulatory element-binding protein-2 (SREBP-2) regulation of human prostasin gene expression. *Biochem Biophys Res Commun.* 346(4):1245–1253.

14. Chen M, Chen LM, Chai KX (2006). Androgen regulation of prostasin gene expression is mediated by sterol-regulatory element-binding proteins and SLUG. *Prostate.* 66(9):911–920.

15. Tuyen DG, Kitamura K, Adachi M, Miyoshi T, Wakida N, Nagano J, Nonoguchi H, Tomita K (2005). Inhibition of prostasin expression by TGF-beta1 in renal epithelial cells. *Kidney Int.* 67(1):193–200.

16. Chen LM, Chai KX (2012). PRSS8 (protease, serine, 8). *Atlas Genet Cytogenet Oncol Haematol.*

17. Sun G, Qin J, Qiu Y, Gao Y, Yu Y, Deng Q, Zhong M (2009). Microarray analysis of gene expression in the ovarian cancer cell line HO-8910 with silencing of the ZNF217 gene. *Mol Med Rep.* 2(5):851–855.

18. Sun M, Nie F, Wang Y, Zhang Z, Hou J, He D, Xie M, Xu L, De W, Wang Z, Wang J (2016). LncRNA HOXA11-as promotes proliferation and invasion of gastric cancer by scaffolding the chromatin modification factors PRC2, LSD1, and DNMT1. *Cancer Res.* 76(21):6299–6310.
19. Wu L, Gong Y, Yan T, Zhang H (2020). LINP1 promotes the progression of cervical cancer by scaffolding EZH2, LSD1, and DNMT1 to inhibit the expression of KLF2 and PRSS8. *Biochem Cell Biol.* 98(5):591–599.
20. Yu JX, Chao L, Chao J (1995). Molecular cloning, tissue-specific expression, and cellular localization of human prostasin mRNA. *J Biol Chem.* 270(22):13483–13489.
21. Yu JX, Chao L, Chao J (1994). Prostasin is a novel human serine proteinase from seminal fluid. Purification, tissue distribution, and localization in prostate gland. *J Biol Chem.* 269(29):18843–18848.
22. Kyte J, Doolittle RF (1982). A simple method for displaying the hydropathic character of a protein. *J Mol Bio.* 157(1):105–132.
23. Rawlings ND, Barrett AJ (2013). Chapter 559 — Introduction: Serine Peptidases and Their Clans. In *Handbook of Proteolytic Enzymes (Third Edition)*, Rawlings ND, Salvesen G (eds.), Academic Press, 2491–2523.
24. Chen LM, Skinner ML, Kauffman SW, Chao J, Chao L, Thaler CD, Chai KX (2001). Prostasin is a glycosylphosphatidylinositol-anchored active serine protease. *J Biol Chem.* 276(24):21434–21442.
25. Pieper U, Webb BM, Dong GQ, Schneidman-Duhovny D, Fan H, Kim SJ, Khuri N, Spill YG, Weinkam P, Hammel M, Tainer JA, Nilges M, Sali A (2014). ModBase, a database of annotated comparative protein structure models and associated resources. *Nucleic Acids Res.* 42(Database issue):D336–D346.
26. Chen LM, Chai JC, Liu B, Strutt TM, McKinstry KK, Chai KX (2021). Prostasin regulates PD-L1 expression in human lung cancer cells. *Biosci Rep.* 41(7):BSR20211370.
27. Tans G, Janssen-Claessen T, Rosing J, Griffin JH (1987). Studies on the effect of serine protease inhibitors on activated contact factors. Application in amidolytic assays for factor XIIa, plasma kallikrein and factor XIa. *Eur J Biochem.* 164(3):637–642.
28. Steen Burrell KA, Layzer J, Sullenger BA (2017). A kallikrein-targeting RNA aptamer inhibits the intrinsic pathway of coagulation and reduces bradykinin release. *J Thromb Haemost.* 15(9):1807–1817.

29. Chen LM, Hodge GB, Guarda LA, Welch JL, Greenberg NM, Chai KX (2001). Down-regulation of prostasin serine protease: A potential invasion suppressor in prostate cancer. *Prostate.* 48(2):93–103.
30. Shipway A, Danahay II, Williams JA, Tully DC, Backes BJ, Harris JL (2004). Biochemical characterization of prostasin, a channel activating protease. *Biochem Biophys Res Commun.* 324(2):953–963.
31. Rickert KW, Kelley P, Byrne NJ, Diehl RE, Hall DL, Montalvo AM, Reid JC, Shipman JM, Thomas BW, Munshi SK, Darke PL, Su HP (2008). Structure of human prostasin, a target for the regulation of hypertension. *J Biol Chem.* 283(50):34864–34872.
32. Spraggon G, Hornsby M, Shipway A, Tully DC, Bursulaya B, Danahay H, Harris JL, Lesley SA (2009). Active site conformational changes of prostasin provide a new mechanism of protease regulation by divalent cations. *Protein Sci.* 18(5):1081–1094.

Chapter 5

The Structure, the Function, and
the Regulation

5.1 The structure

The molecular framework of life is the Central Dogma, which dictates the transfer of genetic information from the genes in the DNA to the RNA transcripts, and then to the proteins encoded by the messenger RNA. The contemporary definition of a gene also includes those that do not encode a protein but terminal RNA molecules, such as ribosomal RNA, transfer RNA, and the many newly discovered varieties of non-coding RNA. In viruses, the genome can be DNA or RNA. The DNA is not chemically inactive, and the bases can be modified as a mechanism of epigenetic regulation for the accessibility of the nucleobases, which contain the genetic information. The nucleobases and the phosphodiester backbone of the DNA can also be chemically damaged, leading to mutations. However, nothing has been reported on the DNA having a biological function beyond storing genetic information.

On the contrary, the 2'-hydroxyl group in the RNA can be deprotonated to become an oxyanion to carry out nucleophilic attacks. These RNA molecules are called ribozymes, as in ribonucleic acid enzymes. The ribosomal peptidyl-transferase function is attributed to the ribosomal RNA of the large subunit, and a very complex higher-ordered structure is the key to forming the ribosomal peptidyl-transferase center (PTC). The ability to carry the genetic information in the nucleobase sequence and serve as a ribozyme, gave RNA the recognition as the likely origin for the text-coded self-replicating form of life.

The limited reaction repertoire with the RNA enzymes using a single choice of the 2'-hydroxyl group as the mechanism yielded to the far more versatile and complex protein world of life today. The repertoire of 20 amino acids with side chains of a full spectrum of biochemical properties, including non-polar hydrophobic, polar, acidic, and basic, gives proteins the ability to fold into all kinds of three-dimensional structures and the choice of more reactive groups. Protein structures are also dynamic and can change in response to changes in the environment to carry out a different function. Learning the structure of a protein in its fine details is essential to understanding the functions of that protein, such as the active site of a proteolytic enzyme. A proper functional analysis of the protein of interest requires the preparation of the protein to a good degree of purity and quantity. In the efforts of obtaining large quantities of pure proteins for such biochemical characterization, the phenomenon of protein crystallization was observed and used as a standard of demonstrating purity.

The first protein crystals observed were from hemoglobins of worms and fish in the mid-1800s. Chicken ovalbumin was crystallized in the late 1800s, followed by the classic enzymes from porcine or bovine pancreas in the 1920s, earning the researchers, Sumner and Northrop, Nobel prizes. The protein crystals are obviously not in their native form in the aqueous cellular context but can still preserve a natural state to allow a proper investigation of the structure. The method of choice for studying protein structures in a crystal was X-ray crystallography, an art perfected by Linus Pauling who established the five rules in 1929 for predicting and rationalizing the crystal structures of ionic compounds, known as Pauling's rules.

X-Ray crystallography generates diffraction patterns of a protein in the crystal. Each atom in a protein molecule is surrounded by a cloud of electrons and these electrons diffract the X-ray to form a unique electron density map that is recorded by a detector. The diffracted patterns by all atoms of a protein can be analyzed *in silico* to generate a 3-dimensional (3-D) image of the protein, as a way of seeing the protein structure at the atomic level as if the protein structure is examined under a very high-resolution microscope.

In 1951, Pauling and others proposed the α-helix and β-sheet as the main structural motifs in the protein secondary structures using models of amino acids and the peptide bond[1]. The work earned Pauling a Nobel Prize in 1954 "for his research into the nature of the chemical bond and its application to the elucidation of the structure of complex substances". Pauling also made significant contributions in the resolution of the double-helical DNA structure using X-ray crystallography.

In 2008, an atomic structure of prostasin was resolved by Rickert and colleagues[2]. A prostasin crystal was formed using a recombinant human prostasin (r-prostasin) made in *E. coli* cells after multiple purification, refolding, and activation procedures. Overall, the crystal structure of the prostasin protease heavy chain is similar to other serine proteases such as having two beta barrel-like subdomains, four disulfide bonds, and a catalytic triad formed by His85, Asp134, and Ser238, which correspond to His57, Asp102, and Ser195 in chymotrypsin's catalytic triad.

The naturally occurring human prostasin would have a total of 12 cysteines. Two were mutated to aid the crystallization and another two, located in the light chain and the GPI-anchor signal region, were excluded, leaving only eight cysteines for the four disulfide bonds in the crystal structure of the recombinant prostasin protein being studied. One of the mutated cysteines is Cys154 which would have formed a disulfide bond with the cysteine in the light chain. The second mutated cysteine is Cys203 which is not conserved among serine proteases and would have formed a disulfide with Cys306 in the carboxyl-terminal region. This disulfide bond could orient the prostasin active site toward the surface of the cell, rendering the catalytic site more accessible or allowing it to co-localize with its substrates.

Prior to the crystallization of prostasin, in 2004, Shipway and colleagues[3] outlined a comprehensive substrate specificity profile of prostasin following a study using position screening substrate libraries. They reported the following substrate preferences for the prostasin serine protease. Prostasin does not auto-activate itself due to the unfavorable isoleucine residue at the P1' site in the zymogen cleavage site

(PQAR↓ITGG). Prostasin prefers basic residues in the P4 position of a substrate. This is supported by the crystal structure of prostasin showing Glu129 interacting with the substrate at the P4 position. Prostasin prefers histidine, lysine, or arginine in the P3 position of a substrate. This could be suggested by the crystal structure of prostasin, in which Gly130, Pro214, and His215 line out the S3 subsite and can accommodate residues with long side chains in the P3 position but may restrict charged residues. Prostasin prefers lysine or arginine in the P1 position of a substrate, and this is determined by Asp232 sitting at the bottom of the S1 pocket, shown in the crystal structure of prostasin.

The tertiary structure of prostasin has a blocked S1 site by a loop containing residues 258–262 (WGDAC). A similar blocked S1 site also exists in other serine proteases such as α1-tryptase, granzyme K, prostate kallikrein (in stallion seminal plasma), and thrombin (Na⁺ free or mutant forms).

The prostasin serine protease activity is regulated by divalent cations. This can be supported by the crystal structure of prostasin with the presence of divalent calcium cation, detailed further in another study.

In 2009, Spraggon and colleagues[4] resolved the crystal structures of r-prostasin in various forms and further revealed the finer structural information on the prostasin protein. They used a non-glycosylated recombinant human prostasin made in the SF9 insect cells. The r-prostasin studied in the crystal form only had the heavy chain. Several variant forms were studied. One had mutated cysteines at 122 and 170. One had a deletion of the hydrophobic carboxyl-terminal sequence (38 amino acid residues) including the GPI-anchor signal to aid crystallization but contained a stretch of 10 histidines as a tag for affinity purification. Four types of crystal were created, including the prostasin apo form, prostasin with the inhibitor d-FFR chloromethyl ketone, prostasin with calcium ion, and prostasin with the serine protease inhibitor aprotinin. Analysis of the four types of crystal suggested that the prostasin S1 pocket is closed but opens upon stimulation by ligands which shift the blocking loop. The S1 pocket closure-and-opening involving the blocking loop, especially without an apparent allosterical activation/inactivation by distal sites, is rather unique to prostasin and could be a mechanism for prostasin protease activity regulation *in vivo* with the changes of divalent cation concentrations under different physiological or pathophysiological conditions.

The crystal structure of prostasin and calcium ion is the same as the apo form except the Ca^{2+} is in the S1 site-blocking loop (residues 215–219, WGDAC) at the bottom of the S1 site interacting with Asp189, preventing substrate entry. The calcium binding may serve as an inhibitory mechanism to the prostasin protease. The Ki of calcium is determined to be 1.15 mM[3], which is below the plasma Ca^{2+} concentration at 2.1–2.6 mM. Prostasin may not be active in the blood, but active in tissues and cells where the calcium concentration is low.

In addition to these atomic-level prostasin structural variations that separate prostasin from other trypsin-like serine protease, a unique feature of the prostasin protein is its GPI anchor which tethers prostasin to the apical side of the epithelial cell surface[5]. The GPI anchor is known to concentrate in cholesterol-rich microdomains of the plasma membrane, also known as the lipid rafts[6]. Release of the GPI-anchored prostasin in a soluble form is mediated by endogenous phospholipases or by proteolytic shedding[7,8].

5.2 The function

Prostasin is the only serine protease anchored to the plasma membrane via a glycosylated-phosphatidylinositol (GPI) lipid complex and expressed in all epithelial cells with a well-established biochemical and physiological function of regulating the ENaC activity. Another GPI-anchored serine protease is testisin/PRSS21, but only expressed in the testis[9].

The human prostasin protein was first discovered and purified from human seminal fluid. The complete biochemical characterization of the purified human prostasin yielded the partial amino acid sequence to enable the design of degenerate oligonucleotides used to clone its cDNA, which in turn enabled the cloning of its gene. The human prostasin gene *PRSS8* is located on chromosome 16p11.2, while the human testisin gene *PRSS21* is at 16p13.3. The ENaC activation function of prostasin awaited the cloning of its homologue from the frog Xenopus using expression cloning to screen for genes that increased the amiloride-sensitive ENaC current in Xenopus oocytes. The frog homologue was named channel-activating protease-1 (CAP-1)[10].

Prostasin was later confirmed to activate ENaC by proteolytically cleaving the ENaC subunits in mammalian epithelial cells[11]. Its existence as a GPI-anchored membrane serine protease opened a new field of study in the serine protease-activated ENaC modulation of extracellular fluid volume and electrolyte homeostasis. Understanding of the structure and membrane localization of prostasin as an extracellular membrane-anchored active serine protease also provided the clues for identifying other candidate protein substrates, which included transmembrane receptors of the receptor tyrosine kinase (RTK) family[12] and the toll-like receptor (TLR) family[13]. Prostasin also interacts with type II transmembrane extracellular serine proteases, matriptase/PRSS14/ST14[14], and hepsin/TMPRSS1[15] in a membrane-localized proteolytic activation network in the epithelial cells. The substrates and inhibitors of prostasin will be described further in later chapters.

Whereas the crystallography studies provided a good volume of information with experimental support from additional studies, the crystallized recombinant prostasin was not in the membrane-anchored form. Another common approach in the study of protein structure-function relationship is to produce variants with amino acid residue changes in the key positions via site-directed mutagenesis in the gene or cDNA coding for the protein. The variants employed in the X-ray crystallography studies of the prostasin heavy chain were for the purpose of facilitating crystallization. For serine proteases, the most relevant variant in a functional study is an alanine replacement of the active-site serine. In theory, the change is minimal in effect on the overall three-dimensional structure of the protease but removes the serine side chain required for the protease function. The variant is often referred to as the "protease-dead" mutant and is very useful to addressing if the proteolytic activity is directly involved or required for a biological function attributed to the protease.

A study conducted on the protease-dead mouse prostasin homologue, named mCAP1, with an alanine replacement of the active-site serine (S238A) gave an unexpected result — the proteolytic activity of the mouse prostasin/mCAP1 was not required for ENaC activation.

This unexpected result was further validated with two additional variants H85A and D134A, changing the other two residues, histidine or aspartic acid in the catalytic triad, to an alanine. Neither had an impact on the mCAP1 in its involvement in ENaC activation. A triple mutant variant with all three catalytic triad residues changed to alanine also had no effect. A variant mCAP1 lacking the GPI-anchor, i.e., a secreted form, failed to activate the ENaC[16]. The results of the protease-dead mCAP1 variants capable of ENaC activation as efficiently as the wild-type mCAP1 would suggest that this function of mCAP1/prostasin/Prss8 does not require the protease activity, or in other words, is protease-independent. It is often further inferred from such results on a protease that there are additional functional domains. This is indeed the case for the type II transmembrane extracellular serine protease matriptase/ST14/PRSS14, with a significantly larger extracellular domain (ECD) than that of the prostasin's. The matriptase ECD contains a sea urchin sperm protein, Enterokinase and Agrin (SEA) domain, two C1r/s, Uegf and Bone morphogenic protein (CUB) domains, four low density lipoprotein receptor (LDLR) domains, and the serine protease domain (SP domain)[17,18]. In the prostasin heavy chain, its entirety is an ECD, no other recognizable domains have been identified by way of sequence homology or experimental evidence. It must be emphasized that such protease-dead variants are not naturally occurring, and these results could represent the cellular response to the imposition of such a variant, especially when over-expressed. One mechanism could be a perturbation of the protease-inhibitor balance that may lead to an enhancement of the activity of another protease which shares the substrate specificity with the wild-type of the inactivated protease[19].

The investigation of the natural substrates of prostasin as a membrane-anchored extracellular protease is greatly challenged by the difficulty associated with creating a proper "test tube" for such experiments. Unlike working with secreted serine proteases which can be done entirely in a test tube and some like trypsin which can be purchased by the buckets, membrane proteases require the membrane context. For the *in vitro* investigations of the substrates and signaling pathways of such membrane-associated proteases, it is necessary to use tissue-cultured cells expressing the endogenous and/or recombinant proteases and their substrates (candidates). It is nearly impossible to rule out an intermediate step involving another protease or a co-factor, even when the introduction of a protease is associated with a cleavage or functional phenotype, unless a protease-substrate complex can be captured. This has not been achieved for a serine protease.

5.3 The regulation

The function of a protease is to perform proteolytic cleavage on its substrates. However, not all proteases are created equal in terms of their physiological roles. Among the serine proteases, the most iconic is the bovine pancreatic trypsin, discovered in 1876 by Wilhelm Kühne, who isolated it by rubbing the pancreas with glycerin and named it as such with the Ancient Greek word for rubbing. Trypsin's main function is digestion of dietary proteins to smaller peptides, which are then broken down to amino acids by other proteases to be absorbed in the intestine. Even in this tissue environment with a dietary protein digestion function of seemingly the brute force kind, the proteolytic activity of the trypsin serine protease must be regulated. Uncontrolled proteases in any tissue environment will cause damages.

The regulation of a protease's function can be at the levels of gene expression, pro-enzyme activation, protease activity modulation by acidity or ionic strength, protease activity inhibition by inhibitors, and compartmentalization to limit the access to their substrates. At the level of gene expression, a protease may be restricted to certain tissues or cell types. A good example is the testis-specific testisin/PRSS21, which is closely related to prostasin in gene and protein structures. Proteases are synthesized as zymogens and would require a proteolytic activation step to enable the final functional conformation, this is true for trypsin and for prostasin. The proteolytic action of a protease is mediated by a nucleophilic attack on the carbonyl group of the scissile bond being cleaved, involving an oxyanion. In the case of serine proteases, the oxyanion is the deprotonated serine side chain in the active site. It is clear that the pH and ionic strengths in the immediate environment of the protease would have an impact on the protease activity, this is true for trypsin and for prostasin as well.

In addition to the digestive function, a whole host of other functions have been attributed to trypsin in a broad range of physiological and pathophysiological conditions. Transcription regulation and pro-enzyme activation can control when and where the enzyme is to be active, but the active enzyme must be neutralized when its function is fulfilled in the spatial and temporal manner. Trypsin is inhibited by the equally iconic α1-antitrypsin, a major plasma protein with levels of 0.9–2.0 g/L in a healthy individual and rising to 4–5 fold higher in an acute inflammation and infection. The increased amount of α1-antitrypsin is critical for neutralizing neutrophil elastase, believed to be the true target enzyme of the inhibitor. α1-Antitrypsin belongs to the serpin class of serine protease inhibitors that act as a suicide substrate, allowing the cleavage of the inhibitor protein by the protease but not the dissociation of its amino-terminal fragment from the enzyme, irreversibly inhibiting the enzyme. For prostasin, a serpin-class serine protease inhibitor, protease nexin-1 (PN-1), has been identified as its cognate irreversible inhibitor via the formation of a covalent complex with the active prostasin[5,20]. Additionally, reversible inhibitors of the prostasin serine protease have also been identified, including hepatocyte growth factor activator inhibitors 1 and 2 (HAI-1 and HAI-2)[21,22].

The term "limited proteolysis" was used to describe the cleavage of some possible scissile bonds within a substrate polypeptide but not all, and the perfect example would be the proteolytic activation of a pro-enzyme, in which only the activation bond is cleaved but not anywhere else in the enzyme itself. It is also used in a different sense to describe the timely control of a protease's action on a substrate, and the perfect example is the inhibition of the blood coagulation cascade serine proteases by their cognate protease inhibitors. The definitive natural substrate of prostasin should be considered unknown even though the presence of prostasin in a cellular and an *in vivo* setting has been associated with physiological as well as protein cleavage phenotypes, as discussed above. Nonetheless the current candidate proteolytic substrates of prostasin, such as the ENaC subunits, members of the RTK family, and TLR4 are all examples of limited proteolysis. Not all sequences matching the substrate requirements in these candidate substrates are cleaved by prostasin. Another mechanism of regulating the protease activity of prostasin toward a candidate substrate is compartmentalization. Prostasin is believed to concentrate in the plasma membrane lipid microdomains, known as the lipid rafts, because of the GPI anchor. The composition of lipid rafts may change in a disease condition, resulting in an abnormal protein distribution and aggregation and an interaction of a candidate substrate with prostasin.

The natural upstream prostasin activator should also be considered as unknown. Matriptase is suggested to be an activating enzyme upstream of prostasin in the epidermis[14], while prostasin is also suggested to be an activating enzyme upstream of matriptase in intestine epithelial cells[23]. The difference is that matriptase can autoactivate its own zymogen but prostasin cannot autoactivate. Hepsin is suggested to be an upstream activator for prostasin, but not vice versa[15]. A recent report suggested that TMPRSS13 can also act as an activating protease upstream of prostasin[24]. In gene knockout experiments, germline inactivation of the mouse *Prss8* gene (encoding prostasin) is associated with embryonic lethality but germline inactivation of the mouse *Prss14* gene (encoding matriptase) permits development to term and birth, despite the death of the neonatal pups due to dehydration from the defective skin. In classical genetics, these phenotypic differences in the gene knockout experiments would place prostasin upstream of matriptase, although the molecular pathways may be unrelated to the proteolytic activation of the zymogens.

Currently, there is strong evidence that prostasin and matriptase are always co-expressed in the epithelial cells[25]. This would be the basis to support prostasin and matriptase as a pair of reciprocal co-activating enzymes regulating each other's activity in various physiological processes relating to epithelial cell proliferation and differentiation. The two enzymes are sorted into different cellular compartments at the terminal differentiation state, preventing unnecessary proteolytic events. In cancers of the B lymphocytes, a rather significant amount of matriptase is expressed[26] but no prostasin expression can be seen at all. However, it is possible that the exosomal prostasin protein can disseminate and travel to the sites of cancerous B lymphocytes to activate the matriptase on those B cells under certain conditions. These observations are also examples of regulation via differential cellular compartmentalization, herein, different cells.

References

1. Pauling L, Corey RB, Branson HR (1951). The structure of proteins; two hydrogen-bonded helical configurations of the polypeptide chain. *Proc Natl Acad Sci USA.* 37(4):205–211.
2. Rickert KW, Kelley P, Byrne NJ, Diehl RE, Hall DL, Montalvo AM, Reid JC, Shipman JM, Thomas BW, Munshi SK, Darke PL, Su HP (2008). Structure of human prostasin, a target for the regulation of hypertension. *J Biol Chem.* 283(50):34864–34872.
3. Shipway A, Danahay H, Williams JA, Tully DC, Backes BJ, Harris JL (2004). Biochemical characterization of prostasin, a channel activating protease. *Biochem Biophys Res Commun.* 324(2):953–963.
4. Spraggon G, Hornsby M, Shipway A, Tully DC, Bursulaya B, Danahay H, Harris JL, Lesley SA (2009). Active site conformational changes of prostasin provide a new mechanism of protease regulation by divalent cations. *Protein Sci.* 18(5):1081–1094.
5. Chen LM, Skinner ML, Kauffman SW, Chao J, Chao L, Thaler CD, Chai KX (2001). Prostasin is a glycosylphosphatidylinositol-anchored active serine protease. *J Biol Chem.* 276(24):21434–21442.
6. Sangiorgio V, Pitto M, Palestini P, Masserini M (2004). GPI-anchored proteins and lipid rafts. *Ital J Biochem.* 53(2):98–111.
7. Iwashita K, Kitamura K, Narikiyo T, Adachi M, Shiraishi N, Miyoshi T, Nagano J, Tuyen DG, Nonoguchi H, Tomita K (2003). Inhibition of prostasin secretion by serine protease inhibitors in the kidney. *J Am Soc Nephrol.* 14(1):11–16.
8. Verghese GM, Gutknecht MF, Caughey GH (2006). Prostasin regulates epithelial monolayer function: Cell-specific Gpld1-mediated secretion and functional role for GPI anchor. *Am J Physiol Cell Physiol.* 291(6):C1258–C1270.
9. Hooper JD, Nicol DL, Dickinson JL, Eyre HJ, Scarman AL, Normyle JF, Stuttgen MA, Douglas ML, Loveland KA, Sutherland GR, Antalis TM (1999). Testisin, a new human serine proteinase expressed by premeiotic testicular germ cells and lost in testicular germ cell tumors. *Cancer Res.* 59(13):3199–3205.

10. Vallet V, Chraibi A, Gaeggeler HP, Horisberger JD, Rossier BC (1997). An epithelial serine protease activates the amiloride-sensitive sodium channel. *Nature*. 389(6651):607–610.

11. Bruns JB, Carattino MD, Sheng S, Maarouf AB, Weisz OA, Pilewski JM, Hughey RP, Kleyman TR (2007). Epithelial Na+ channels are fully activated by furin- and prostasin-dependent release of an inhibitory peptide from the gamma-subunit. *J Biol Chem*. 282(9):6153–6160.

12. Chen M, Chen LM, Lin CY, Chai KX (2008). The epidermal growth factor receptor (EGFR) is proteolytically modified by the Matriptase-Prostasin serine protease cascade in cultured epithelial cells. *Biochim Biophys Acta*. 1783(5):896–903.

13. Uchimura K, Hayata M, Mizumoto T, Miyasato Y, Kakizoe Y, Morinaga J, Onoue T, Yamazoe R, Ueda M, Adachi M, Miyoshi T, Shiraishi N, Ogawa W, Fukuda K, Kondo T, Matsumura T, Araki E, Tomita K, Kitamura K (2014). The serine protease prostasin regulates hepatic insulin sensitivity by modulating TLR4 signalling. *Nat Commun*. 5:3428.

14. Netzel-Arnett S, Currie BM, Szabo R, Lin CY, Chen LM, Chai KX, Antalis TM, Bugge TH, List K (2006). Evidence for a matriptase-prostasin proteolytic cascade regulating terminal epidermal differentiation. *J Biol Chem*. 281(44):32941–32945.

15. Chen M, Chen LM, Lin CY, Chai KX (2010). Hepsin activates prostasin and cleaves the extracellular domain of the epidermal growth factor receptor. *Mol Cell Biochem*. 337(1–2):259–266.

16. Andreasen D, Vuagniaux G, Fowler-Jaeger N, Hummler E, Rossier BC (2006). Activation of epithelial sodium channels by mouse channel activating proteases (mCAP) expressed in Xenopus oocytes requires catalytic activity of mCAP3 and mCAP2 but not mCAP1. *J Am Soc Nephrol*. 17(4):968–976.

17. Lin CY, Anders J, Johnson M, Sang QA, Dickson RB (1999). Molecular cloning of cDNA for matriptase, a matrix-degrading serine protease with trypsin-like activity. *J Biol Chem*. 274(26):18231–18236.

18. Takeuchi T, Shuman MA, Craik CS (1999). Reverse biochemistry: Use of macromolecular protease inhibitors to dissect complex biological processes and identify a membrane-type serine protease in epithelial cancer and normal tissue. *Proc Natl Acad Sci USA*. 96(20):11054–11061.

19. Chen M, Fu YY, Lin CY, Chen LM, Chai KX (2007). Prostasin induces protease-dependent and independent molecular changes in the human prostate carcinoma cell line PC-3. *Biochim Biophys Acta*. 1773(7):1133–1140.

20. Chen LM, Zhang X, Chai KX (2004). Regulation of prostasin expression and function in the prostate. *Prostate*. 59(1):1–12.

21. Fan B, Wu TD, Li W, Kirchhofer D (2005). Identification of hepatocyte growth factor activator inhibitor-1B as a potential physiological inhibitor of prostasin. *J Biol Chem*. 280(41):34513–34520.

22. Coote K, Atherton-Watson HC, Sugar R, Young A, MacKenzie-Beevor A, Gosling M, Bhalay G, Bloomfield G, Dunstan A, Bridges RJ, Sabater JR, Abraham WM, Tully D, Pacoma R, Schumacher A, Harris J, Danahay H (2009). Camostat attenuates airway epithelial sodium channel function in vivo through the inhibition of a channel-activating protease. *J Pharmacol Exp Ther*. 329(2):764–774.

23. Buzza MS, Martin EW, Driesbaugh KH, Désilets A, Leduc R, Antalis TM (2013). Prostasin is required for matriptase activation in intestinal epithelial cells to regulate closure of the paracellular pathway. *J Biol Chem*. 288(15):10328–10337.

24. Murray AS, Hyland TE, Sala-Hamrick KE, Mackinder JR, Martin CE, Tanabe LM, Varela FA, List K (2020). The cell-surface anchored serine protease TMPRSS13 promotes breast cancer progression and resistance to chemotherapy. *Oncogene*. 39(41):6421–6436.

25. List K, Hobson JP, Molinolo A, Bugge TH (2007). Co-localization of the channel activating protease prostasin/(CAP1/PRSS8) with its candidate activator, matriptase. *J Cell Physiol*. 213:237–245.

26. Gao L, Liu M, Dong N, Jiang Y, Lin CY, Huang M, Wu D, Wu Q (2013). Matriptase is highly upregulated in chronic lymphocytic leukemia and promotes cancer cell invasion. *Leukemia*. 27(5):1191–1194.

Chapter 6

The Roles in Physiology and Pathophysiology — An Overview

In a whole body or a cell where a protein is expressed under normal conditions in a state of homeostasis, it is very challenging to assign a functional role to the protein. An illness or a disease is a perturbation of the homeostasis and the result of the body, an organ, or a tissue taking a hit. The hit can be an inborn molecular defect, a microorganism, or a chemical, while the effects can be transient, or long-term. In the diseased state, the manifested pathophysiology is accompanied by corresponding changes of the relevant molecules, either qualitatively or quantitatively. In the early days and years of studying the human pathophysiology, the most common point of entry was the analysis of the most easily obtained bodily fluids such as the blood and the urine, or the solid waste (stool) to examine the changes of metabolites as a readout or report of what systems or parts of the body were malfunctioning.

The Online Mendelian Inheritance in Man (OMIM) catalogs human genes and genetic disorders. The first hereditary human disorder to be described was alkaptonuria[1,2], by Sir Archibald Garrod in 1902. The clinical manifestations include urine turning dark on exposure, black ochronotic pigmentation of cartilage and collagenous tissues, and arthritis, most prominent in the spine. The defect enzyme in the patients was identified in 1958 to be homogentisate 1,2-dioxygenase (HGD; E.C.1.13.11.5)[3].

The molecular genetic defect was determined following the mapping of the disease gene[4,5], encoding homogentisate 1,2-dioxygenase, a

63

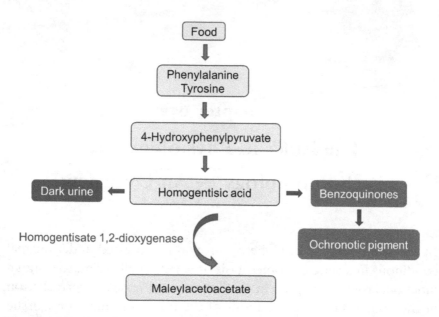

Figure 6-1. Simplified pathways of alkaptonuria. The excess homogentisic acid discharged in the urine will turn dark brown upon oxidization, whereas the by-product benzoquinone acetate forms melanin-like polymers that deposit in tissues.

long 94 years later in 1996[6]. A loss of this gene and the enzyme leaves the metabolic processing of the aromatic amino acids, phenylalanine and tyrosine, short at the step of homogentisic acid, which is subsequently diverted to form benzoquinone acetic acid. The latter forms polymers that resemble the skin pigment melanin and can be deposited in tissues, causing the clinical manifestations described above[7,8] (Figure 6-1).

The lesson, as well as the wisdom that we could draw from this example and many that followed, is that the cellular or system homeostasis must be perturbed by a "challenge" to effect a molecular change for the functional role of a protein to be revealed. In the tissue culture setting, this can be achieved by drug or chemical treatments, the introduction of a gene (in the form of a cDNA plasmid) coding for the protein of interest for an over-expression, or an inhibitory RNA to silence the endogenous gene coding for that protein of interest. In other words, a gain-of-function or loss-of-function condition is artificially created to bring about an associative phenotype, from which the pathophysiological role of the protein is inferred and the normal physiological role is implicated. In the whole-body setting, the gain-of-function or loss-of-function condition can also be created in animal models by introducing a transgene via microinjection into the one-cell embryo or via a viral vector, or knocking out the endogenous gene in the germline or in a tissue- or cell-specific manner.

No human condition has been cataloged in the OMIM for the prostasin gene. Many suggested physiological or pathophysiological roles of prostasin were delineated from studies using animal models, e.g., laboratory mice and rats. Mice and rats share similar biological features with humans. Both models can be genetically engineered to either over-express a human gene, or knockout the counterpart of a human gene, more often in the mouse. Mice and rats are small in size, and they are easy to maintain in a relatively large number by a research laboratory or a commercial facility. In addition, they have a lifetime of 2–3 years which is a short timeframe for studying biological mechanisms of genes and monitoring disease progression over a developmental course.

6.1 Extracellular fluid volume and blood pressure regulation

The *in vivo* function of prostasin was first explored in 2003 by Wang and colleagues[9] in the Wistar rats (Harlan Sprague Dawley, Indianapolis, IN) by introducing the human prostasin gene (cDNA) via an adenovirus vector. The rationale of this study was that prostasin had been demonstrated in epithelial cell lines *in vitro* to activate the epithelial sodium channel (ENaC), a key player in the regulation of the body's extracellular fluid volume and electrolyte balance.

Delivery of the human prostasin-expressing adenovirus into the tail vein of rats resulted in a sustained blood pressure increase for 3–4 weeks. Interestingly, on Day 3 after the gene delivery, the plasma aldosterone level was increased before a noticeable increase of the blood pressure on Day 5, suggesting that the higher level of aldosterone may have caused an increase of the extracellular fluid volume, leading to an increase in the blood pressure. In addition, the plasma renin activity was decreased and the renal excretion of Na^+, K^+, and kallikrein increased. Aldosterone is a steroid hormone made in the zona glomerulosa of the adrenal gland cortex and secreted into the blood. Analysis of the tissue distribution of human prostasin in rat tissues, after the adenovirus-mediated prostasin gene delivery, revealed prostasin expression in the adrenal glands. It is possible that the ectopically expressed prostasin in the adrenal glands up-regulated aldosterone production either directly or indirectly by unknown mechanisms. The exact role of prostasin in this rat model is not clear, the study points to some potential mechanisms of cross-talking by the renin-angiotensin-aldosterone and kallikrein-kinin systems, both involved in blood pressure and electrolyte homeostasis. Whether prostasin regulates aldosterone production or vice versa was investigated in the ensuing years with inconsistent findings.

Several transgenic mouse models were created by silencing the prostasin gene in specific tissues for investigating prostasin regulation on the ENaC activity.

In 2005, Leyvraz and colleagues[10] reported that neonatal mice die within 60 hours after birth if the prostasin gene is silenced in the epidermis. Interestingly, the cause of death is severe dehydration due to tissue architectural defects of the skin without affecting the ENaC activity.

In 2010, Planès and colleagues[11] observed that mice with a prostasin deficiency in the alveolar epithelium of the lung had a reduced ability to clear the alveolar fluid in response to an acute volume overload via the mechanism of regulating the ENaC sodium transport.

In 2014, Malsure and colleagues[12] studied the phenotypes of mice with the prostasin expression silenced in the colon and suggested that prostasin participates in the ENaC-mediated sodium transport in the colon *in vivo*, and this regulation is more pronounced when the renin-angiotensin-aldosterone system is activated in the afternoon during the day.

In 2022, Ehret and colleagues[13] suggested that prostasin is dispensable from the mouse kidney based on the studies of mice lacking prostasin expression in the kidney tubular cells.

Is prostasin a regulator of the ENaC? It appeases that prostasin may serve different roles in different tissues. This will be discussed in further detail in later chapters.

6.2 The immune system and inflammation

Transgenic mice over-expressing a human prostasin transgene for gain-of-function studies were created in the Chao lab at the Medical University of South Carolina (MUSC) during 2003–2005. Independent transgenic lines were generated via intra-embryo microinjection of a linearized plasmid DNA containing the full-length human prostasin cDNA driven by the Rous sarcoma virus long-terminal repeat (RSV-LTR) promoter. The confirmed transgenic mice would have a chromosomally integrated human prostasin cDNA for anticipated ubiquitous expression. These mice were subjected to a study where a bladder inflammation was induced via intraperitoneal injection of the bacterial lipopolysaccharides (LPS)[14]. The expression of the endogenous mouse prostasin was significantly reduced by ~70% during the first 18 hours of the inflammation response. Accordingly, the expression of several key cytokines was up-regulated. However, the transgenic mice with a human prostasin over-expression had shown a reduced cytokine expression in response to the LPS treatment. This model allowed the investigation of both loss-of-function and gain-of-function with the prostasin gene under the challenge by a clinically relevant inflammatory agent. The inflammation down-regulates the endogenous mouse *Prss8* gene, with or without the chromosomally integrated human PRSS8 transgene (cDNA) in two independent transgenic lines and in the parent control line. Pathophysiologically, the event of the mouse *Prss8* gene expression down-regulation may be a prerequisite for the induction of the cytokine interferon gamma (IFNγ) and the inducible nitric oxide synthase (iNOS). The expression of the human PRSS8 transgene (cDNA) is unaffected by the inflammatory agent and represents a gain-of-function in the same event, with the phenotype of attenuating the IFNγ induction in the transgenic lines and the iNOS induction in the transgenic line with a robust PRSS8 transgene (cDNA) expression.

In 2014, in a loss-of-function study, Uchimura and colleagues[15] generated a mouse model with a targeted *Prss8* gene deletion in the liver and reported that the up-regulation of the inflammatory cytokines, in response to an LPS challenge, was potentiated by the prostasin expression silencing.

In 2021, Sugitani and colleagues[16] generated a mouse model in which the *Prss8* gene was deleted in the intestinal epithelial cells. With the cell-specific silencing of prostasin's expression, the mucosa of the intestinal tract was more vulnerable to developing dextran sodium sulfate (DSS)-induced colitis. These studies firmly suggested a prostasin function in the innate immune response.

Investigations in the animals in loss- or gain-of-function models are the most direct and powerful to reveal the associative *in vivo* phenotypes of the gene of interest, but the detailed molecular pathways would require a cell-based approach. When the pathophysiological event is elicited in a well-studied pathway, the candidate interactive molecules could be identified and tested by further cellular and biochemical means. In inflammation and the innate immune response, when the challenging agent is the bacterial LPS, a candidate interactive and mediating molecule would be the toll-like receptor 4 (TLR4). Further analysis did provide evidence for TLR4 to be a natural transmembrane protein substrate for prostasin, a GPI-anchored extracellular proteolytically active membrane serine protease.

6.3 Embryo implantation and placenta development

The loss-of-function animal models discussed above involved the inactivation of the mouse *Prss8* gene in a tissue- or cell-specific manner. We have already learned that the OMIM does not have a single entry of hereditary disorder associated with a human *PRSS8* gene mutation. It was learned from efforts to create a germline mouse *Prss8* gene knockout (KO) in the Chao lab in 2005 at the MUSC, that the *Prss8* gene is required in early embryonic development. This was deduced from a lack of homozygote *Prss8* KO litters among the 130 offspring from crosses of the hemizygotes with one *Prss8* KO allele (Chai, unpublished results, University of Central Florida), defying the anticipated Mendelian distribution. This lethal phenotype was also observed by Hummler and colleagues[17] in 2013 with a more detailed examination of the *in utero* embryos genotyped as the homozygote *Prss8* KO. The molecular mechanistic roles of prostasin in the embryonic development at the steps of embryo implantation and placental development will be discussed in a later chapter.

6.4 Epidermis maturation

In 2005, Leyvraz and colleagues[10] created a conditional *Prss8* KO model in which the prostasin gene was disrupted only in the epidermis. The *K14-Cre* mice were crossed with hemizygote mice in which exons 3–5 were flanked by the *loxP* sites in one copy of the *Prss8* gene while the other copy was deleted. The K14-Cre is expressed specifically in the skin to mediate the complete elimination of *Prss8* exons 3–5 via loxP recombination only in the skin. In the offspring, the skin cells would have a "homozygous" knockout of *Prss8*. These mice survived through the embryonic stages but died quickly within 60 hours after birth due to dehydration, as the result of a severely underdeveloped neonatal skin.

6.5 Glucose and lipid metabolism

In 2021, Sekine and colleagues[18] reported that mice with a human PRSS8 transgene (cDNA) over-expression, specifically in the liver, had improved glucose tolerance and serum cholesterol level when fed with a high-fat diet. Those mice also had reduced hepatic lipid accumulation and reduced hepatic steatosis. The liver specific PRSS8 transgene (cDNA) expression was achieved with the use of the mouse albumin gene promoter.

6.6 Cancer

Many lines of evidence indicated that prostasin expression is down-regulated in many tumors of an epithelial origin, with the first example being cancers of the prostate, reported in 2001 by Chen and colleagues[19]. Cancer cells arise from multiple genetic hits accumulated during proliferation in a stepwise progression, as postulated by Carl Nordling in the early 1950s[20]. In 1971, Alfred Knudson proposed the "two-hit hypothesis" after studying retinoblastomas in sporadic cases versus the inherited cases[21]. The two-hit hypothesis concerns the inactivation of genes that serve as tumor suppressors to counter the effects of oncogenes that drive and promote oncogenesis. The loss of one tumor suppressor allele is ordinarily insufficient to allow the tumors to develop but a second hit that takes away the remaining allele sets forth the full course of tumorigenesis. The putative tumor-suppressor gene RB1 postulated by Knudson to have such a role and fate in retinoblastoma was cloned in 1986[22]. In the early 2000s, Peter Jones added to the two-hit hypothesis with epigenetic silencing being a potential mechanism for the hits[23]. Epigenetic silencing of the human *PRSS8* gene by DNA hypermethylation and histone deacetylation was first observed in invasive human prostate and breast cancer cell lines.

It was not clear if the down-regulation of prostasin in the epithelial cancers was causal or merely an effect. In 2019, Bao and colleagues[24] created a mouse KO model with the *Prss8* gene inactivated in the intestinal tract. The tissue-specific absence of prostasin was associated with spontaneous intestinal inflammation and a high frequency of adenoma development with age. These observations are consistent with a tumor suppressor role for prostasin.

References

1. Garrod AE (1902). The incidence of alkaptonuria: A study in chemical individuality. *The Lancet*. 160(4137):1616–1620.
2. Garrod AE (1908). The Croonian Lectures on inborn errors of metabolism, lecture II Alkaptonuria. *The Lancet*. 2:73–79.
3. La Du BN, Zannoni VG, Laster L, Seegmiller JE (1958). The nature of the defect in tyrosine metabolism in alkaptonuria. *J Biol Chem*. 230(1):251–260.
4. Pollak MR, Chou YH, Cerda JJ, Steinmann B, La Du BN, Seidman JG, Seidman CE (1993). Homozygosity mapping of the gene for alkaptonuria to chromosome 3q2. *Nat Genet*. 5(2):201–204.

5. Janocha S, Wolz W, Srsen S, Srsnova K, Montagutelli X, Guénet JL, Grimm T, Kress W, Müller CR (1994). The human gene for alkaptonuria (AKU) maps to chromosome 3q. *Genomics.* 19(1):5–8.

6. Fernández-Cañón JM, Granadino B, Beltrán-Valero de Bernabé D, Renedo M, Fernández-Ruiz E, Peñalva MA, Rodríguez de Córdoba S (1996). The molecular basis of alkaptonuria. *Nat Genet.* 14(1):19–24.

7. Introne WJ, Perry M, Chen M (2003). Alkaptonuria. In *GeneReviews®* *[Internet]*, Adam MP, Everman DB, Mirzaa GM, Pagon RA, Wallace SE, Bean LJH, Gripp KW, Amemiya A (eds.), Seattle (WA): University of Washington, Seattle, 1993–2022.

8. Zatkova A, Ranganath L, Kadasi L (2020). Alkaptonuria: Current perspectives. *Appl Clin Genet.* 13:37–47.

9. Wang C, Chao J, Chao L (2003). Adenovirus-mediated human prostasin gene delivery is linked to increased aldosterone production and hypertension in rats. *Am J Physiol Regul Integr Comp Physiol.* 284(4):R1031–R1036.

10. Leyvraz C, Charles RP, Rubera I, Guitard M, Rotman S, Breiden B, Sandhoff K, Hummler E (2005). The epidermal barrier function is dependent on the serine protease CAP1/Prss8. *J Cell Biol.* 170(3):487–496.

11. Planès C, Randrianarison NH, Charles RP, Frateschi S, Cluzeaud F, Vuagniaux G, Soler P, Clerici C, Rossier BC, Hummler E (2010). ENaC-mediated alveolar fluid clearance and lung fluid balance depend on the channel-activating protease 1. *EMBO Mol Med.* 2(1):26–37.

12. Malsure S, Wang Q, Charles RP, Sergi C, Perrier R, Christensen BM, Maillard M, Rossier BC, Hummler E (2014). Colon-specific deletion of epithelial sodium channel causes sodium loss and aldosterone resistance. *J Am Soc Nephrol.* 25(7):1453–1464.

13. Ehret E, Jäger Y, Sergi C, Mérillat AM, Peyrollaz T, Anand D, Wang Q, Ino F, Maillard M, Kellenberger S, Gautschi I, Szabo R, Bugge TH, Vogel LK, Hummler E, Frateschi S (2022). Kidney-specific CAP1/Prss8-deficient mice maintain ENaC-mediated sodium balance through an aldosterone independent pathway. *Int J Mol Sci.* 23(12):6745.

14. Chen LM, Wang C, Chen M, Marcello MR, Chao J, Chao L, Chai KX (2006). Prostasin attenuates inducible nitric oxide synthase expression in lipopolysaccharide-induced urinary bladder inflammation. *Am J Physiol Renal Physiol.* 291(3):F567–F577.

15. Uchimura K, Hayata M, Mizumoto T, Miyasato Y, Kakizoe Y, Morinaga J, Onoue T, Yamazoe R, Ueda M, Adachi M, Miyoshi T, Shiraishi N, Ogawa W, Fukuda K, Kondo T, Matsumura T, Araki E, Tomita K,

Kitamura K (2014). The serine protease prostasin regulates hepatic insulin sensitivity by modulating TLR4 signalling. *Nat Commun.* 5:3428.

16. Sugitani Y, Nishida A, Inatomi O, Ohno M, Imai T, Kawahara M, Kitamura K, Andoh A (2020). Sodium absorption stimulator prostasin (PRSS8) has an anti-inflammatory effect via downregulation of TLR4 signaling in inflammatory bowel disease. *J Gastroenterol.* 55(4):408–417.

17. Hummler E, Dousse A, Rieder A, Stehle JC, Rubera I, Osterheld MC, Beermann F, Frateschi S, Charles RP (2013). The channel-activating protease CAP1/Prss8 is required for placental labyrinth maturation. *PLoS One.* 8(2):e55796.

18. Sekine T, Takizawa S, Uchimura K, Miyazaki A, Tsuchiya K (2021). Liver-specific overexpression of prostasin attenuates high-fat diet-induced metabolic dysregulation in mice. *Int J Mol Sci.* 22(15):8314.

19. Chen LM, Hodge GB, Guarda LA, Welch JL, Greenberg NM, Chai KX (2001). Down-regulation of prostasin serine protease: A potential invasion suppressor in prostate cancer. *Prostate.* 48(2):93–103.

20. Nordling CO (1953). A new theory on cancer-inducing mechanism. *Br J Cancer.* 7(1):68–72.

21. Knudson AG Jr (1971). Mutation and cancer: statistical study of retinoblastoma. *Proc Natl Acad Sci USA.* 68(4):820–823.

22. Friend SH, Bernards R, Rogelj S, Weinberg RA, Rapaport JM, Albert DM, Dryja TP (1986). A human DNA segment with properties of the gene that predisposes to retinoblastoma and osteosarcoma. *Nature.* 323(6089):643–646.

23. Jones PA, Baylin SB (2002). The fundamental role of epigenetic events in cancer. *Nat Rev Genet.* 3(6):415–428.

24. Bao Y, Guo Y, Yang Y, Wei X, Zhang S, Zhang Y, Li K, Yuan M, Guo D, Macias V, Zhu X, Zhang W, Yang W (2019). PRSS8 suppresses colorectal carcinogenesis and metastasis. *Oncogene.* 38(4):497–517.

Chapter 7

Prostasin in the Kidney — Regulating the ENaC Activity

Five thousand years ago, recorded in 黄帝内经 (Huang Di Nei Jing), an ancient Chinese medical text was the observation "if too much salt is used in food, the pulse hardens, tears make their appearance and the complexion changes"[1]. It means that an alteration of the sodium (Na+) homeostasis would affect a person's blood pressure.

In humans, the primary function of the kidney is to maintain the body's extracellular fluid volume and electrolyte balance via regulating the sodium (Na+) homeostasis. The functional unit of the kidney is the nephron. Each nephron is about 30–55 mm long, consisting of segments of Bowman's capsule enclosing the glomerular capillary vessels, the proximal tubule, the descending limb of loop, loop of Henle, the ascending limb of loop, the distal tubule, and the collecting duct. There are about one million nephrons in each human kidney. The kidneys fulfill the functions of filtration, reabsorption, secretion, and excretion. The blood from the circulation enters the glomerular capillary vessels at the afferent arteriole and soluble blood components can enter the lumen of the Bowman's capsule. This step is filtration and the glomeruli in the kidneys can filter a massive 180 liters of blood per day. Blood components that do not enter the lumen, i.e., 80% of the plasma volume that enter the afferent arteriole, travel back into the circulation through the efferent arteriole. The filtration step removes the chemical wastes from the blood and these eventually go out with the urine. However, not all filtered soluble contents are waste. Thus, in the tubular segments, the next step is reabsorption, in which water is recovered by the cotransport of glucose and sodium. For the 20% of filtrates from the glomerulus, over 19% of the fluid is reabsorbed in the remainder of the nephron. Therefore, more than 99% of the plasma entering the kidney returns to the systemic circulation and less than 1% of the volume is excreted to the external environment.

The blood pressure is sensed and regulated by baroreceptors which are mechanical sensors located within the blood vessels. Baroreceptors receive mechanical stimulation from the blood vessel, such as stretching, due to the change in the blood pressure and convey the stimulation to the brain for blood pressure adjustment by changing the peripheral vascular resistance and cardiac output.

Regulation of the peripheral vascular resistance can be achieved by angiotensin II, a vasoconstrictor in the renin-angiotensin system (RAS). Renin, an aspartic protease, is released from the juxtaglomerular cells of the kidney to the blood circulation, where it converts angiotensinogen released from the liver to angiotensin I. The latter is further converted to angiotensin II by the angiotensin-converting enzyme (ACE), a metalloprotease produced by the endothelium of pulmonary blood vessels. In addition to directly increasing blood vessel contraction to increase the peripheral vascular resistance, angiotensin II also stimulates aldosterone production and secretion. The steroid hormone aldosterone released from the zona glomerulosa in the adrenal gland cortex acts on the aldosterone target tissues/cells to increase the epithelial sodium channel (ENaC) expression and promote sodium retention in the extracellular space. This will lead to an increase in the blood pressure. Aldosterone stimulates Na^+ reabsorption by regulating Na^+ transport via increasing the transcription of the ENaC genes in the kidney, and in turn increasing the ENaC number at the apical membrane of the collecting duct, with a probability of more open channels.

In clinical cases, gain-of-function mutations in the ENaC subunit genes are found in Liddle's syndrome, an inherited autosomal-dominant disease. The mutations in the ENaC genes disabled the ENaC degradation pathway, resulting in more ENaC on the membrane surface, an increased Na^+ reabsorption, and increased extracellular fluid volume. Patients with Liddle's syndrome usually have salt-sensitive hypertension[2]. On the contrary, lost-of-function mutations in the ENaC subunit genes are found in pseudohypoaldosteronism type 1 (PHA1) condition, an inherited autosomal-recessive disease[3]. The mutations in the ENaC genes disable the ENaC function, and the outcome is an inability or a reduced ability of Na⁺ reabsorption in the kidney. Patients with the PHA1 condition usually have salt-wasting hypotension despite having high levels of aldosterone in the blood. These monogenic mutations underscore the significance of the ENaC in body sodium homeostasis and blood pressure regulation[4,5].

Sodium reabsorption through the ENaC in the distal nephron is the first and rate-limiting step in transepithelial sodium transport[6]. Serine proteases had long been implicated in the regulation of ENaC activity[7,8]. In a study using the isolated toad urinary bladder, the reversible serine protease inhibitor aprotinin, which was used in the purification of prostasin from human seminal plasma, was shown to decrease the short-circuit current (SCC). The SCC is measured by using an Ussing chamber, devised by the Danish zoologist and physiologist Hans Henriksen Ussing in 1946. It is used for measuring epithelial membrane properties such as ion transport with the SCC as an indicator of the net ion transport across an epithelium, in the form of either a live and native tissue, such as the isolated toad urinary bladder, or a monolayer of cells grown on a permeable support[9].

Amiloride is a drug used to treat high blood pressure, as a potassium-sparing diuretic. Amiloride blocks the ENaC, reducing the absorption of the sodium ion and the excretion of the potassium ion. Serine proteases with biochemical properties similar to that of the glandular kallikrein were postulated as candidate proteolytic activators of the epithelial sodium channel. The search for the true channel-activating serine proteases by biochemical means encountered a major problem, in that the candidate enzymes activate but also degrade the amiloride-sensitive sodium channel.

In search of the endogenous ENaC-activating serine proteases, Vallet and colleagues[10] performed a functional complementation assay using Xenopus oocytes. The A6 Xenopus kidney epithelial cells, established from the principal cells of the collecting ducts, were treated with aldosterone. The mRNAs were then isolated from the treated cells and subjected to a size fractionation over sucrose-gradient centrifugation.

The size fractionated A6 mRNAs were co-injected with the ENaC sub-unit cRNAs (prepared from the cDNAs) and expressed in the oocytes. An increase of ~40% of the amiloride-sensitive sodium current was observed in the oocyte co-expressing the αβγENaC cRNA and the frac-tionated A6 mRNA in the 1–2-kilobase (kb) size range. Subsequently, a cDNA library was made using the 1–2-kb fractionated mRNA and screened by co-injection of the cRNA from pools of the cDNA and the αβγENaC cRNAs. In the ensuing rounds of dissecting the pools of cRNAs with such a turnkey-operation functional complementation assay, one clone was identified and isolated based on its ability to induce an increase of the amiloride-sensitive sodium current by ~3 fold.

The isolated cDNA clone is 1,340 base-pairs (bp) long, containing a 987-nucleotide (nt) open-reading frame which encodes a predicted protein with 329 amino acid residues. This protein is named xCAP1 for Xenopus channel-activating protease 1. xCAP1 shares an amino acid sequence identity with the human serine protease prostasin at 53% and has a carboxyl-terminal hydrophobic domain reminiscent of the glycosylphosphatidylinositol (GPI)-anchor signal for a post-trans-lational modification. The GPI anchor would bring the xCAP1 to the apical cell surface of the highly polarized A6 cells to interact with the αβγENaC proteins at the same membrane location. Further, the ENaC activation property of the xCAP1 protein was confirmed by co-expression of xCAP1 with either the Xenopus αβγENaC (xENaC) or the rat αβγENaC (rENaC) in Xenopus oocytes. Once again, the amiloride-sensitive sodium current was increased in both co-expression experiments and most likely by an increase in the overall ENaC open probability[11,12]. The A6 Xenopus kidney epithelial cells were stimulated with aldosterone before the mRNA isolation and size-fractionation. The regulation of prostasin/xCPA1 expression by aldosterone became a research focus of many researchers in the ensuing years. This subject is discussed in later chapters.

The xCAP1 mRNA was found by northern blot analysis to be highly expressed in the kidney, intestine, stomach, skin, and lung, where ENaC is expressed as well. This seminal work opened a new research area and raised a new hypothesis that the ENaC activity is regulated by a membrane-anchored extracellular serine protease. An xCAP1 membrane localization in close proximity with the ENaC is deemed critical for ENaC activation[13]. A mutant xCAP1 without the membrane anchorage and secreted into the culture medium did not activate the ENaC. However, this may be due to the lack of accessibility of the secreted xCAP1 in the medium to the ENaC on the membrane, as the secreted xCPA1 may be too diluted to have a critical mass in contact with the ENaC to proteolytically activate it.

In 2000, Vuagniaux and colleagues[14] set out to identify the mammalian orthologue of xCAP1 in the mpkCCDc14 mouse kidney cell line of the collecting duct origin. Based on the sequence of xCAP1, degenerate oligonucleotides were designed and used for amplifying a 512-bp cDNA fragment by means of RT-PCR from the mpkCCDc14 cell mRNA. Then, the technique of "rapid amplification of cDNA ends" (5'-RACE and 3'-RACE) (Life Technologies) was used to determine both ends of the extended cDNA sequence. Finally, a 1,768-bp cDNA fragment was amplified and confirmed by DNA sequencing. Similar to the xCAP1 cDNA, this mouse cDNA encodes a 339-residue protein which shared an 80% sequence homology with the human prostasin protein. This new protein is designated as mCAP1 for mouse channel-activating protease 1 and the new protein is also presumed to be tethered to the membrane via a GPI anchor. The mCAP1 cDNA was transcribed *in vitro* and the cRNA was injected into Xenopus oocytes along with ENaC cRNAs from the Xenopus (xENaC), or rat (rENaC), or human (hENaC) for functional analysis. The amiloride-sensitive Na^+ current was increased. It was suggested that mCAP1 is the mouse counterpart of prostasin in humans and mCAP1 appears to increase the overall open probability of ENaC, i.e., activating the pre-existing channels located in the plasma membrane since the number of ENaC on the cell surface did not change in response to the expression of mCAP1.

The expression of mCAP1 was investigated by northern blot analysis and found to be mostly present in the kidney, lung, colon, and salivary glands, with co-expression of the ENaC α-subunit. Further analysis on the microdissected mouse nephron, by means of RT-PCR, revealed that the proximal tubule, including the convoluted and straight terminal portions, expressed the highest amounts of mCAP1. The expression of mCAP1 was also detected in the cortical ascending limbs of Henle's loop and the cortical collecting duct. Medullary ascending limbs of Henle's loop, the inner medullary collecting duct, and the distal convoluted tubules express a rather low level of mCAP1. Aldosterone works on the distal nephron in the aldosterone responsive segment and regulates the rate of Na[+] reabsorption[15,16]. The distal nephron consists of the distal convoluted tubules and collecting ducts, all of which respond to aldosterone stimulation. The presence of prostasin expression in the kidney proximal tubules, which are non-aldosterone responsive, suggested a local mode of modulation of the ENaC by prostasin.

In 2001, soon after the cloning of mCAP1, Adachi and colleagues[17] cloned a full-length prostasin cDNA from the rat kidney by means of RT-PCR, 3'-RACE, and 5-RACE, using degenerate primers based on the human prostasin amino acid sequence. The cDNA clone contains a 1,029-bp coding region which encodes a 342-residue protein with a presumed GPI anchor. A 223-bp 5'-noncoding region and a 956-bp 3'-noncoding region are also included in the cloned full-length cDNA. Similar to the human prostasin, a potential N-glycosylation site is located at Asn159, and the three amino acid residues constituting the catalytic triad are identified as His85, Asp134, and Ser238 in the deduced amino acid sequence of the rat prostasin.

The rat prostasin shares a 77% sequence identity with the human prostasin and is predominantly expressed in the kidney cortex and medulla, but less in the prostate, lung, colon, stomach, and skin, as determined by means of northern blot analysis and RT-PCR. Micro-dissection of the rat collecting tubules and determination by RT-PCR, indicated that the prostasin mRNA is expressed in the cortical collecting duct (CCD), the outer medullary collecting ducts (OMCD), and the inner medullary collecting ducts (IMCD). A functional study indicated that the rat prostasin can activate the rat $\alpha\beta\gamma$ENaC in Xenopus oocytes. Interestingly, this study did not support the hypothesis that prostasin increases single-channel open probability of the ENaC (as in the case of xCAP1 and mCAP1), nor that prostasin proteolytically activates a fraction of the "silent channels" on the Xenopus oocyte surface. Rather, it was speculated that prostasin increases the number of functional ENaC in the plasma membrane. Nonetheless, this study on the rat prostasin provided further support to the hypothesis that mCAP1, xCAP1, and human prostasin are orthologues, as proposed by Vuagniaux and colleagues[14] in 2000.

Thus far, the functional analysis of ENaC activation by CAP1/prostasin was performed in Xenopus oocytes. In 2002, Narikiyo and colleagues investigated whether prostasin regulates sodium balance *in vivo* in mammals[18]. Prostasin expression and Na+ transport were evaluated in the M-1 mouse cortical collecting duct cells, in rats infused with aldosterone via a subcutaneously implanted osmotic minipump, as well as in patients with primary aldosteronism. Aldosterone treatment increased prostasin mRNA expression in the M-1 cells and its protein secretion in the culture medium. The ^{22}Na uptake was increased accordingly in the treated M-1 cells.

In the aldosterone-infused rats and in patients with primary aldosteronism, the urinary excretion of prostasin was increased. Adrenalectomy normalized the patients' plasma aldosterone and reverted the high urinary excretion of prostasin, suggesting an aldosterone regulation in the excretion of prostasin likely via enhancing the prostasin expression in the kidney, in addition to the previously demonstrated functions of aldosterone such as increasing the ENaC number and the open probability of the channels.

In 1999, Masilamani and colleagues[16] applied dietary sodium salt restriction or aldosterone infusion to Sprague-Dawley rats to increase the aldosterone level in the blood circulation. Consequently, the abundance of the ENaC α-subunit was increased in the collecting principal cells at the apical plasma membrane and the molecular weight of the ENaC γ-subunit was reduced from 85 kDa to 70 kDa, suggesting a proteolytic cleavage of the subunit presumably just beyond the first membrane-spanning region. The newly identified CAP1 was one of the candidates for the cleavage. In 2007, Bruns and colleagues[19] confirmed that a cleavage of the ENaC γ-subunit by prostasin removes the inhibitory tract peptide to fully activate the ENaC. In 2015, Zachar and colleagues[20] reported that the cleaved ENaC γ-subunit, possibly by prostasin, was seen only in human urine samples of proteinuria.

Aldosterone increases prostasin expression in humans with primary aldosteronism and apparently, there is a fraction of prostasin being secreted in the urine independent of the sodium intake or the aldosterone level in the blood[18,21]. The secreted prostasin could be the source of the enzyme responsible for ENaC activation in other segments of the renal tubules, an example of paracrine regulation as opposed to the autocrine regulation where both ENaC and prostasin are expressed in the same cell on the apical surface. The exosomes may be a way for the secreted prostasin to retain its membrane anchorage, which is required for ENaC activation in such a paracrine mechanism[13,22].

As we mentioned in the previous chapter, in 2003, Wang and colleagues[23] gave a single injection of adenovirus harboring the human prostasin cDNA into the Wistar rats and monitored the rat blood pressure for four weeks. Rat adrenal glands are not known for expressing prostasin but the imposed expression of a recombinant human prostasin in rat adrenal glands may have triggered aldosterone expression and secretion either directly or indirectly via unknown pathways, resulting in the elevated aldosterone level in the rat plasma two days before the onset of hypertension. Aldosterone, then, may have increased the ENaC expression and promoted Na^+ reabsorption in the kidney. In addition, the recombinant human prostasin in the rat kidney may have activated ENaC and increased Na^+ reabsorption as well. All of these may have contributed to the increased blood pressure in the rats. Prostasin stimulation of aldosterone production in the adrenal gland was later confirmed by Ko and colleagues[24] in 2010. In that study, the H295R human adrenocortical cell line was used as a model. Unexpectedly, the prostasin-induced aldosterone synthesis did not involve the proteolytic activity of prostasin.

As can be seen from all the studies described above, the role of prostasin in sodium homeostasis and its relationship with aldosterone are highly complex with much known but even more unknown. Prostasin could also have a role in ENaC activation via activating matriptase, a type-II transmembrane serine protease with the alias CAP3, for channel-activating protease 3. Matriptase/CAP3 expression in the PC-3 human prostate cancer cells can be dramatically induced at both the transcription and translation levels by the expression of a protease-dead prostasin variant, in which the active-site serine was replaced by an alanine[25]. This molecular mechanism may perhaps offer a way to reconcile some phenotypic observations made for the protease-dead prostasin variant introduced in cultured cells or transgenic animals[26]. For example, a protease-dead variant mCAP1 with all three catalytic triad amino acid residues replaced, retained its ability to activate the ENaC, as we have discussed in Chapter 5.

Reference

1. Ilza Veith (2002). Section 10 — Treatise on the Five Viscera in Relation to Their Part in Perfecting Life. In *The Yellow Emperor's Classic of Internal Medicine*. University of California Press, Berkerley, United States.
2. Shimkets RA, Warnock DG, Bositis CM, Nelson-Williams C, Hansson JH, Schambelan M, Gill JR Jr, Ulick S, Milora RV, Findling JW (1994). Liddle's syndrome: Heritable human hypertension caused by mutations in the beta subunit of the epithelial sodium channel. *Cell.* 79(3):407–414.
3. Chang SS, Grunder S, Hanukoglu A, Rösler A, Mathew PM, Hanukoglu I, Schild L, Lu Y, Shimkets RA, Nelson-Williams C, Rossier BC, Lifton RP (1996). Mutations in subunits of the epithelial sodium channel cause salt wasting with hyperkalaemic acidosis, pseudohypoaldosteronism type 1. *Nat Genet.* 12(3):248–253.
4. Hansson JH, Nelson-Williams C, Suzuki H, Schild L, Shimkets R, Lu Y, Canessa C, Iwasaki T, Rossier B, Lifton RP (1995). Hypertension caused by a truncated epithelial sodium channel gamma subunit: Genetic heterogeneity of Liddle syndrome. *Nat Genet.* 11(1):76–82.
5. Boiko N, Kucher V, Stockand JD (2015). Pseudohypoaldosteronism type 1 and Liddle's syndrome mutations that affect the single-channel properties of the epithelial Na+ channel. *Physiol Rep.* 3(11):e12600.
6. Canessa CM, Schild L, Buell G, Thorens B, Gautschi I, Horisberger JD, Rossier BC (1994). Amiloride-sensitive epithelial Na+ channel is made of three homologous subunits. *Nature.* 367(6462):463–467.
7. Orce GG, Castillo GA, Margolius HS (1980). Inhibition of short-circuit current in toad urinary bladder by inhibitors of glandular kallikrein. *Am J Physiol.* 239(5):F459–F465.
8. Lewis SA, Clausen C (1991). Urinary proteases degrade epithelial sodium channels. *J Membr Biol.* 122(1):77–88.
9. Clarke LL (2009). A guide to Ussing chamber studies of mouse intestine. *Am J Physiol Gastrointest Liver Physiol.* 296(6):G1151–G1166.

10. Vallet V, Chraibi A, Gaeggeler HP, Horisberger JD, Rossier BC (1997). An epithelial serine protease activates the amiloride-sensitive sodium channel. *Nature*. 389(6651):607–610.

11. Chraïbi A, Vallet V, Firsov D, Hess SK, Horisberger JD (1998). Protease modulation of the activity of the epithelial sodium channel expressed in Xenopus oocytes. *J Gen Physiol*. 111(1):127–138.

12. Caldwell RA, Boucher RC, Stutts MJ (2004). Serine protease activation of near-silent epithelial Na+ channels. *Am J Physiol Cell Physiol*. 286(1):C190–C194.

13. Vallet V, Pfister C, Loffing J, Rossier BC (2002). Cell-surface expression of the channel activating protease xCAP-1 is required for activation of ENaC in the Xenopus oocyte. *J Am Soc Nephrol*. 13(3):588–594.

14. Vuagniaux G, Vallet V, Jaeger NF, Pfister C, Bens M, Farman N, Courtois-Coutry N, Vandewalle A, Rossier BC, Hummler E (2000). Activation of the amiloride-sensitive epithelial sodium channel by the serine protease mCAP1 expressed in a mouse cortical collecting duct cell line. *J Am Soc Nephrol*. 11(5):828–834.

15. Duc C, Farman N, Canessa CM, Bonvalet JP, Rossier BC (1994). Cell-specific expression of epithelial sodium channel alpha, beta, and gamma subunits in aldosterone-responsive epithelia from the rat: Localization by in situ hybridization and immunocytochemistry. *J Cell Biol*. 127(6 Pt 2):1907–1921.

16. Masilamani S, Kim GH, Mitchell C, Wade JB, Knepper MA (1999). Aldosterone-mediated regulation of ENaC alpha, beta, and gamma subunit proteins in rat kidney. *J Clin Invest*. 104(7):R19–R23.

17. Adachi M, Kitamura K, Miyoshi T, Narikiyo T, Iwashita K, Shiraishi N, Nonoguchi H, Tomita K (2001). Activation of epithelial sodium channels by prostasin in Xenopus oocytes. *J Am Soc Nephrol*. 12:1114–1121.

18. Narikiyo T, Kitamura K, Adachi M, Miyoshi T, Iwashita K, Shiraishi N, Nonoguchi H, Chen LM, Chai KX, Chao J, Tomita K (2002). Regulation of prostasin by aldosterone in the kidney. *J Clin Invest*. 109(3): 401–408.

19. Bruns JB, Carattino MD, Sheng S, Maarouf AB, Weisz OA, Pilewski JM, Hughey RP, Kleyman TR (2007). Epithelial Na+ channels are fully activated by furin- and prostasin-dependent release of an inhibitory peptide from the gamma-subunit. *J Biol Chem*. 282(9):6153–6160.

20. Zachar RM, Skjødt K, Marcussen N, Walter S, Toft A, Nielsen MR, Jensen BL, Svenningsen P (2015). The epithelial sodium channel

α-subunit is processed proteolytically in human kidney. *J Am Soc Nephrol.* 26(1):95–106.

21. Olivieri O, Castagna A, Guarini P, Chiecchi L, Sabaini G, Pizzolo F, Corrocher R, Righetti PG (2005). Urinary prostasin: A candidate marker of epithelial sodium channel activation in humans. *Hypertension.* 46(4):683–688.

22. Chen LM, ChaiJC, Liu B, Strutt TM, McKinstry KK, Chai KX (2021). Prostasin regulates PD-L1 expression in human lung cancer cells. *Biosci Rep.* 41(7):BSR20211370.

23. Wang C, Chao J, Chao L (2003). Adenovirus-mediated human prostasin gene delivery is linked to increased aldosterone production and hypertension in rats. *Am J Physiol Regul Integr Comp Physiol.* 284(4):R1031–R1036.

24. Ko T, Kakizoe Y, Wakida N, Hayata M, Uchimura K, Shiraishi N, Miyoshi T, Adachi M, Aritomi S, Konda T, Tomita K, Kitamura K (2010). Regulation of adrenal aldosterone production by serine protease prostasin. *J Biomed Biotechnol.* 2010:793843.

25. Chen M, Fu YY, Lin CY, Chen LM, Chai KX (2007). Prostasin induces protease-dependent and independent molecular changes in the human prostate carcinoma cell line PC-3. *Biochim Biophys Acta.* 1773(7):1133–1140.

26. Andreasen D, Vuagniaux G, Fowler-Jaeger N, Hummler E, Rossier BC (2006). Activation of epithelial sodium channels by mouse channel activating proteases (mCAP) expressed in Xenopus oocytes requires catalytic activity of mCAP3 and mCAP2 but not mCAP1. *J Am Soc Nephrol.* 17(4):968–976.

Chapter 8

Prostasin in the Airways

In the preceding chapter we examined the roles played by prostasin serine protease in the kidney, regulating sodium reabsorption and the extracellular volume, and in turn, the blood pressure. If water can be regarded as the foremost important to living things, oxygen is the immediate next, or perhaps, a co-first. The air supplies oxygen to us, and we take up oxygen by tissues that are in direct contact with the atmospheric oxygen. The tissue with the most open and direct access to the atmospheric oxygen is our skin, with an average of 22 square feet or 2 square meters in its total area. Indeed, we have known for more than 170 years that the skin does take up the atmospheric oxygen, but the amount is near negligible as compared to the respiratory uptake, and the significance of this local oxygen uptake to the skin tissue is not clear. From the front of our eyes, oxygen can also diffuse across the cornea, but the surface area here is even tinier. The only other tissue that is exposed to the atmospheric oxygen, but also the biggest in surface area, is the lung. The average set of human lungs has 480 million alveoli, with a total of 500–800 square feet (50–75 square meters) in surface area!

Ordinarily, the air that we breathe in is almost unfiltered and would carry everything in the air, such as dust particles, pathogens, etc. The interface of the airway tissue to the atmosphere is not dry, quite unlike the air-skin interface, the epidermis. The human airway epithelial surface is covered by a thin layer of airway surface liquid (ASL) serving as the lubricant and a protective coat between the epithelium and the outside environment. This mechanism of protection brings a challenge to the breathing function, thus the ASL needs to be intricately and delicately managed. The ASL volume is regulated to maintain a ~7 μm periciliary liquid layer (PCL) for efficient cilia beating, and a mucus layer sitting atop of the periciliary layer for trapping debris and pathogens[1,2]. The mucus moves from the distal airways to the proximal airways, eventually out of the human body as sputa, finishing the course of removing the trapped particulates.

Sodium transport across the airway epithelium is an important mechanism in the regulation of the ASL volume. The main driving force for this mechanism is the epithelial sodium channel (ENaC) on the epithelial cell membrane. The ENaC absorbs and transfers sodium ions (Na^+) from the extracellular fluid/lumen across the apical membrane into the cytoplasm of the cell. The Na^+ ions are then pumped out of the cytoplasm into the interstitial fluid by the Na^+/K^+ ATPase located on the basolateral membrane. During this process, an osmotic gradient is created, allowing water molecules to passively move into the cell along with Na^+, extruding the fluid out of the alveolar space. On a different path, the cystic fibrosis transmembrane conductance regulator (CFTR), a chloride channel, regulates Cl^- secretion and creates an osmotic pressure to bring water from the inside out to the lumen to hydrate the airways.

At birth, the ENaC activity accounts for the rapid removal of the alveolar fluid to adapt to the gas exchange function in the postnatal life. In adulthood, the ENaC is constitutively active to maintain a thin layer of the ASL or to resolve oedema. An impaired ENaC function in the lungs could thus understandably have severe consequences, as shown by studies in an animal model, in which the α-subunit of the mouse ENaC was inactivated by gene knockout. The mouse dies within 40 hours after birth, due to an inability to remove liquid from the lungs[3].

Each functional unit of the ENaC is formed by the homologous α-, β-, and γ-subunits, and is presented on the apical side of the polarized epithelial cell membrane[4]. The ENaC subunits are encoded by the *SCNN1A*, *SCNN1B*, and *SCNN1G* genes, respectively. The ENaC matures in the Golgi apparatus after a furin cleavage, to remove an inhibitory peptide in the α-subunit before translocating to the apical plasma membrane, a step known as the intrinsic regulation. Therein and after, the ENaC is fully activated to gain the maximum activity at the high open probability, after another proteolytic cleavage to remove an inhibitory peptide in the γ-subunit, a step known as the local extracellular extrinsic regulation. The ENaC can also be extrinsically regulated systemically by hormones such as aldosterone, arginine vasopressin, the atrial natriuretic peptide (ANP), insulin, and endothelin, all of which could affect ENaC expression, intracellular trafficking, or degradation. As human airways do not respond to aldosterone very well, the local regulation of the ENaC activity plays a major role in the lung epithelial cells[5].

To identify serine proteases responsible for ENaC activation in the human airway epithelium, Donaldson and colleagues[6] carried out a homology screening of a human tracheobronchial epithelial cDNA library, in 2002. They first amplified a partial cDNA fragment from the RNA of human tracheobronchial epithelial cells using degenerate primers designed with the deduced amino acid sequence of Xenopus channel-activating protease 1 (xCAP1). Using the partial cDNA as the probe, two positive clones were identified from the human tracheobronchial epithelial cDNA library. These two clones were sequenced and confirmed to be coding for prostasin and TMPRSS2 (transmembrane protease, serine 2). This cloning strategy was essentially based on the assumption that a channel-activating serine protease, homologous to the xCAP1, would be expressed at a reasonable abundance in the lung epithelial cells, where its action is physiologically relevant. To assign a functional role for prostasin or TMPRSS2 in the regulation of ENaC activity in the lung epithelial cells, two additional steps must be taken. First, a "gain of function" study to see if either can perform the task and second, a "loss-of-function" study to see if either is both sufficient but also necessary as the ENaC-activating protease in the lung epithelium. The critical studies addressing these are outlined next.

Functional analysis of these two human serine proteases on ENaC activation was performed by co-expressing the protease and ENaC in Xenopus oocytes followed by two-electrode voltage clamp sodium current measurements. Co-expression of the human prostasin with the rat ENaC (rENaC) or Xenopus ENaC (xENaC) cRNA in the Xenopus oocyte expression system resulted in an ~80% Na$^+$ current increase with rENaC or ~60% Na$^+$ current increase with xENaC. Activation of the

ENaC by prostasin can be completely blocked by adding the serine protease inhibitor aprotinin, suggesting that its extracellular serine protease activity was required for the activation. Interestingly, co-expression of TMPRSS2 with the ENaC in Xenopus oocyte resulted in a completely opposite outcome from that with prostasin. The Na^+ current was decreased by TMPRSS2 when compared to the controls in which only the ENaC was expressed. Further analysis by means of western blotting on the proteins of the total oocyte lysate and the microsomal fractions failed to detect the ENaC protein in the oocytes expressing both the ENaC and TMPRSS2. In addition, aprotinin did not prevent the ENaC loss in the presence of TMPRSS2. It is possible that the reduced Na^+ current was due to the loss of the ENaC protein in the oocytes in the presence of TMPRSS2, but not an apparent pseudo-inhibition function of TMPRSS2 to the ENaC activity. These observations suggest a degradative function of TMPRSS2 on the ENaC.

In situ hybridization analysis localized prostasin mRNA expression in human respiratory epithelial cells lining the airways and submucosal glands, including the nose (upper airways) and the trachea, bronchi, and alveoli (lower airways). In an *in vitro* primary nasal epithelial cell culture system, adding trypsin did not increase the Na^+ current, indicating that the ENaC is fully active with the endogenously expressed serine proteases. However, if the cells were pretreated with aprotinin, trypsin could further increase the Na^+ current. This suggests that the ENaC was always kept open and active under that cell culturing condition, and extra proteases will not activate more ENaC. In addition, inhibitors of proteases may have kept the ENaC activation at a basal level in a steady state. However, if the ASL volume alters for any reason, the balance between serine proteases and their inhibitors in the local ASL environment can be changed as a result, which could have an impact on the ENaC activity[7,8]. The hypothesis that prostasin is the human orthologue of xCAP1 regulating ENaC activity was supported by Donaldson and colleagues.

The research summarized above had established a sufficient functional role for the human prostasin to positively regulate ENaC activity in the lungs while ruling out TMPRSS2 for such an involvement, despite being pulled out by the homology screening looking for the molecular homologue of xCAP1. To provide further evidence that prostasin plays a role in lung fluid balance via regulating ENaC activity, especially to establish that the involvement of prostasin in the regulation of lung epithelial ENaC activity is also necessary, loss-of-function studies were conducted.

In 2010, Planès and colleagues[9] used the conditional Cre-loxP-mediated recombination technique to create a triple-transgenic mouse model lacking the functional full-length prostasin protein in the lung alveolar epithelium in a tissue-specific manner. In the homozygote mice, exons 3–5 of the prostasin gene were edited out along with a frameshift generating a premature termination codon in exon 6. The truncated prostasin protein does not possess a complete catalytic triad and is composed of only 30% of the whole native molecule from the carboxyl terminus. The prostasin gene inactivation was inducible with doxycycline and the knockout event only happens in the mouse alveolar epithelium due to the specific expression of surfactant proteins (SPA and SPC) that drive the expression of the recombinase. The disruption/knockout of the prostasin gene locus in the target cells resulted in a 95% reduction of prostasin expression at the mRNA level.

These knockout mice did not appear to be different in any aspect of the lung anatomy and functions examined, including the structures of the bronchioles, the alveolar ducts, and the alveolar epithelium in the lung, or the water content in the lung. However, the isolated alveolar epithelial cells (AEC) from the prostasin gene knockout mice did not handle the transepithelial Na$^+$ transport very well, with a 40% decrease in the ENaC-mediated sodium currents. A further examination of the basal level of alveolar fluid clearance (AFC) in the mice indicated a 48% reduction as compared with that of the control mice. The results from these loss-of-function studies did not show that prostasin is the only ENaC-activating protease in the lung epithelial cells but a major role in such a capacity is nonetheless assigned to it. Prostasin functions in the lungs were further investigated by modeling the human diseases.

Pulmonary edema, characterized by excess fluid accumulation in the alveolar spaces, is a life-threatening condition resulting from many serious pathophysiological states or diseases such as congestive heart failure (CHF). To evaluate if alveolar fluid clearance (AFC) is compromised in mice under stress and without prostasin expression, experiments using a hydrostatic volume-overload model mimicking pulmonary oedema were carried out. The prostasin knockout mice had a reduced ability in handling Na^+ transport in the lung alveoli, manifested by an increased volume of the alveolar epithelial lining fluid under the challenge of an acute intravascular volume expansion. More important, the AEC lacking prostasin responded much less to a β2-agonist stimulation, which is known to promote airway fluid clearance via β2-adrenergic receptor activation[10]. In addition, without prostasin in the AEC, the intracellular pool of the ENaC protein could reach the apical membrane after the β2-agonist stimulation, but the ENaC does not appear to be fully functional. These studies support the hypothesis that prostasin activates the ENaC in the lung AEC, and that prostasin expression in the AEC is required for the optimal stimulation of AFC by β-agonists.

Prostasin deficiency increases the alveolar epithelial lining fluid accumulation in an experimental model of hydrostatic pulmonary oedema. This *in vivo* animal model study suggested that prostasin is an important and physiologically relevant activator of the ENaC, playing a crucial role in lung fluid balance. Similarly, patients manifesting the autosomal recessive pseudohypoaldosteronism, a rare syndrome of mineralocorticoid resistance due to mutations in the ENaC genes, have no marked impairment in the clearance of lung liquid at birth but develop respiratory illnesses later due to diminished sodium absorption, increased ASL volume, and markedly accelerated rates of mucociliary clearance, resulting in an excessive volume of liquid in the lungs and an increased ASL volume[11–13].

The ASL volume is tightly regulated with the coordination of the Na^+ absorption by the epithelial sodium channel (ENaC) and the Cl^- secretion by the chloride channel, the cystic fibrosis transmembrane conductance regulator (CFTR). An abnormal volume of the ASL is implicated in the pathogenesis of chronic lung diseases such as cystic fibrosis and chronic obstructive pulmonary disease (COPD), whereas mucociliary clearance serves as an indicator of lung health.

In an *in vitro* study using a primary human airway epithelial cell culture (HAEC), it was demonstrated that in a healthy epithelium, the ASL volume is auto-regulated by the ENaC. The equilibrium between proteases and their inhibitors maintains a pool of the ENaC at a near-silent status. In a disease state, e.g., cystic fibrosis (CF), the protease activity can be dysregulated by the ASL volume change, leading to a constitutive proteolytic activation of the ENaC and a pathological Na⁺ hyperabsorption[7,8,14]. In the HAEC culture, prostasin was found on the apical side of the HAEC and secreted from the HAEC in the culture medium, but the secretion was not observed basolaterally. Even though the prostasin protein could be detected at the basolateral membrane of the cells, it is not being activated or correctly processed for secretion. Meanwhile, prostasin can be detected from the sputum of CF patients.

Cystic fibrosis[15] is a genetic disorder that affects multiple organs especially in glands that produce mucus and sweat. Mutations in the *CFTR* gene lead to the development of cystic fibrosis[16]. CF patients have increased ENaC activities, therefore, less airway surface liquid (ASL), causing the mucus buildup to become thick and sticky. The thick mucus can block the lung airways, rendering it increasingly difficult to breathe with frequent infections in the lungs. It was very intriguing that a high dose of the non-steroidal anti-inflammatory drug (NSAID) ibuprofen had a beneficial effect in patients with cystic fibrosis manifesting a mild lung disease, when the NSAID was taken over the long term[17,18]. Such a benefit, however, was not observed in another study[19]. In an *in vitro* study using a human bladder cell culture, prostasin expression was increased by ibuprofen treatment[20]. It would be interesting to investigate if prostasin expression in human airway epithelial cells is up-regulated by ibuprofen as well. However, if a prostasin up-regulation were to be present in patients taking ibuprofen long-term, it may not directly offer an interpretation of the beneficial effects observed in that first study, as the prostasin up-regulation could increase ENaC activation. It would be quite an understatement that prostasin has a plethora of biochemical and physiological functions by interacting with many membrane or secreted proteins. Thus, it is not surprising that in the complex context of drug actions in a disease state, different studies may present different findings. The discrepancy may add to our frustration in the understanding of this versatile membrane serine protease but should also drive our curiosity to ask more questions.

To improve *in vitro* cell culture models for studying ENaC and CFTR functions in regulating the ASL volume, a bronchial culture system was established to mimic the *in vivo* airway epithelial-ASL volume regulation[8]. Ciliated and goblet cells were included in this system to create an organized periciliary liquid layer (PCL) and mucus layer[21]. Confocal microscopy was used to measure the ASL volume. Based on the reported data, both the Na^+ and the Cl^- transports were required to maintain an ASL volume at 7 µm in order to cover the cilia underneath the fluid/mucus. In CF patients, the Cl^- transport is impaired while the Na^+ transport is increased. The imbalance of the Na^+ and Cl^- transports leads to a depleted ASL volume.

Prostasin expression is regulated by the ASL and an abnormal prostasin expression may be responsible for the over-activated ENaC in cystic fibrosis patients, worsening the symptoms. Silencing the prostasin gene in the cystic fibrosis lung cell line reduced the Na^+ current, suggesting that prostasin is a major regulator of the ENaC-mediated Na^+ current in the deltF508 cystic fibrosis epithelium, and prostasin could be a target of therapeutic intervention to alleviate the symptoms of CF patients[22].

Förster resonance energy transfer (FRET) is a method that can be used to measure enzyme-substrate interactions at the distance of intermolecular space on the order ~1–10 nm[23]. The FRET reporters can detect serine proteases in solution or on the cell surface after the lipid modification of the protease to insert it into the outer leaflet of the plasma membrane. By using the ratiometric, peptide-based FRET reporting technique, serine protease activity can be visualized on the cell membrane. It was shown that prostasin's activity was increased on the cell surface of CF patients, lending support to the possibility that a hyperactivity of prostasin increases the ENaC activity, exacerbating the CF conditions[24].

In summary, the ENaC operates as the rate-limiting step for sodium absorption[12,25] and is a critical determinant of the ASL volume. Prostasin serine protease is identified as an activator that cleaves the ENaC γ-subunit and increases the channel open probability of near-silent ENaC[26-28]. Prostasin's regulation on ENaC activity was also supported by a gene-silencing experiment, in which, prostasin gene expression in a CF airway epithelial cell line was silenced by prostasin-specific small interference RNA (siRNA). The Na⁺ conductance was reduced by 75%, underpinning the critical function of prostasin in ENaC regulation[22]. The ASL volume is controlled by active ion transport rather than "passive" physical forces such as surface tension[1,29]. It is not known how the opposing Na⁺ absorptive and Cl⁻ secretory ion transport pathways are coordinately regulated to achieve an ASL volume homeostasis in the normal airways or how they are perturbed in the cystic fibrosis airways. Mice of a triple-transgenic model[30] harboring genes for over-expression of the αβγENaC die within two days after birth, underscoring the importance of precision regulation of ENaC activity.

A high level of the ASL volume was shown to increase the expression of prostasin, which can lead to more proteolytic activation of the ENaC, increases in sodium transport, and a reduction of the ASL volume in a molecular feedback loop. The ASL volume change presents to the cells as a mechanical signal, whereas the induction of prostasin gene expression is a molecular response from inside the nucleus. How then, is a mechanical signal from outside of the cell coupled to a molecular event that far downstream inside? At the moment, the picture is far from clear but some clues with which to move forward can be gathered. The best molecular candidates for mechanosensing and mechanotransduction of signals are membrane proteins, and the key players identified to date include some that are fairly straightforward, the integrins, E-cadherin, and the epidermal growth factor receptor (EGFR). Stiffening of the extracellular matrix has been known to induce integrin clustering, which can crosstalk with EGF-EGFR signaling. The EGFR, and the closely related Her2/ErbB2 can guide cell spreading in response to differences in matrix stiffness via mechanosensing, independent of ligand activation. All these membrane mechanosensing proteins crossed path with prostasin in past research investigations but a detailed potential mechanism awaits an initial delineation. As a matter of fact, the ENaCs are themselves mechanosensing proteins and can be activated by mechanical force variations imposed onto the epithelial cells. However, this can further complicate matters because it will be necessary to peel away the direct mechanical activation of the ENaC from the part played by prostasin in future investigations on mechano-regulation of the ASL equilibrium.

Aerovance, a Bayer spinoff biopharmaceutical company, was developing drugs (trade-named Aerolytic and Pulmolytic) that were mimetics of a serine protease inhibitor, to inhibit prostasin as a way to down-modulate the ENaC in CF patients in the clinical setting. The rationale was based on an estimate that prostasin causes about 80% of the mucus production in CF patients. The project attracted a significant level of funding more than a decade ago. No update is apparently available currently. Additionally, no other therapeutics using prostasin as an agent or a target has seen clinical application at this time. Throughout our discussion of the current knowledge and understanding on the biochemical functions and physiological roles of prostasin, it is clear that an absence of this important membrane serine protease, where it is naturally expressed, is detrimental to living organisms. Too much of prostasin expression paradoxically has similar phenotypes as those produced when prostasin is absent (as in the case of knockouts), at least in the aspects of the epithelial cell tight junction formation and maintenance[20,31]. The challenge in future endeavors will be to find ways to finesse prostasin's quantity and/or activity by delivery as an agent or inhibition as a target *in situ*.

References

1. Tarran R, Grubb BR, Gatzy JT, Davis CW, Boucher RC (2001). The relative roles of passive surface forces and active ion transport in the modulation of airway surface liquid volume and composition. *J Gen Physiol.* 118(2):223–236.
2. Knowles MR, Boucher RC (2002). Mucus clearance as a primary innate defense mechanism for mammalian airways. *J Clin Invest.* 109(5):571–577.
3. Hummler E, Barker P, Gatzy J, Beermann F, Verdumo C, Schmidt A, Boucher R, Rossier BC (1996). Early death due to defective neonatal lung liquid clearance in alpha-ENaC-deficient mice. *Nat Genet.* 12(3):325–328.
4. Canessa CM, Schild L, Buell G, Thorens B, Gautschi I, Horisberger JD, Rossier BC (1994). Amiloride-sensitive epithelial Na+ channel is made of three homologous subunits. *Nature.* 367(6462):463–467.

5. Stokes JB, Sigmund RD (1998). Regulation of rENaC mRNA by dietary NaCl and steroids: Organ, tissue, and steroid heterogeneity. *Am J Physiol.* 274(6):C1699–C1707.

6. Donaldson SH, Hirsh A, Li DC, Holloway G, Chao J, Boucher RC, Gabriel SE (2002). Regulation of the epithelial sodium channel by serine proteases in human airways. *J Biol Chem.* 277(10):8338–8345.

7. Myerburg MM, Butterworth MB, McKenna EE, Peters KW, Frizzell RA, Kleyman TR, Pilewski JM (2006). Airway surface liquid volume regulates ENaC by altering the serine protease-protease inhibitor balance: A mechanism for sodium hyperabsorption in cystic fibrosis. *J Biol Chem.* 281(38):27942–27949.

8. Tarran R, Trout L, Donaldson SH, Boucher RC (2006). Soluble mediators, not cilia, determine airway surface liquid volume in normal and cystic fibrosis superficial airway epithelia. *J Gen Physiol.* 127(5):591–604.

9. Planès C, Randrianarison NH, Charles R-P, Frateschi S, Cluzeaud F, Vuagniaux G, Soler P, Clerici C, Rossier BC, Hummler E (2010). ENaC-mediated alveolar fluid clearance and lung fluid balance depend on the channel-activating protease 1. *EMBO Mol Med.* 2(1): 26–37.

10. Pittet JF, Wiener-Kronish JP, McElroy MC, Folkesson HG, Matthay MA (1994). Stimulation of lung epithelial liquid clearance by endogenous release of catecholamines in septic shock in anesthetized rats. *J Clin Invest.* 94(2):663–671.

11. Kerem E, Bistritzer T, Hanukoglu A, Hofmann T, Zhou Z, Bennett W, MacLaughlin E, Barker P, Nash M, Quittell L, Boucher R, Knowles MR (1999). Pulmonary epithelial sodium-channel dysfunction and excess airway liquid in pseudohypoaldosteronism. *N Engl J Med.* 341(3):156–162.

12. Rossier BC (2004). The epithelial sodium channel: Activation by membrane-bound serine proteases. *Proc Am Thorac Soc.* 1(1):4–9.

13. Katz C, Bentur L, Elias N (2011). Clinical implication of lung fluid balance in the perinatal period. *J Perinatol.* 31(4):230–235.

14. Myerburg MM, McKenna EE, Luke CJ, Frizzell RA, Kleyman TR, Pilewski JM (2008). Prostasin expression is regulated by airway surface liquid volume and is increased in cystic fibrosis. *Am J Physiol Lung Cell Mol Physiol.* 294(5):L932–L941.

15. Anderson DH (1938). Cystic fibrosis of the pancreas and its relation to celiac disease: A clinical and pathologic study. *Am J Dis Child.* 56: 344–399.

16. Ratjen F, Döring G (2003). Cystic fibrosis. *Lancet.* 361(9358):681–689.
17. Konstan MW, Byard PJ, Hoppel CL, Davis PB (1995). Effect of high-dose ibuprofen in patients with cystic fibrosis. *N Engl J Med.* 332(13):848–854.
18. Lands LC, Milner R, Cantin AM, Manson D, Corey M (2007). High-dose ibuprofen in cystic fibrosis: Canadian safety and effectiveness trial. *J Pediatr.* 151(3):249–254.
19. Fennell PB, Quante J, Wilson K, Boyle M, Strunk R, Ferkol T (2007). Use of high-dose ibuprofen in a pediatric cystic fibrosis center. *J Cyst Fibros.* 6(2):153–158.
20. Chai AC, Robinson AL, Chai KX, Chen LM (2015). Ibuprofen regulates the expression and function of membrane-associated serine proteases prostasin and matriptase. *BMC Cancer.* 15:1025.
21. Matsui H, Grubb BR, Tarran R, Randell SH, Gatzy JT, Davis CW, Boucher RC (1998). Evidence for periciliary liquid layer depletion, not abnormal ion composition, in the pathogenesis of cystic fibrosis airways disease. *Cell.* 95(7):1005–1015.
22. Tong Z, Illek B, Bhagwandin VJ, Verghese GM, Caughey GH (2004). Prostasin, a membrane-anchored serine peptidase, regulates sodium currents in JME/CF15 cells, a cystic fibrosis airway epithelial cell line. *Am J Physiol Lung Cell Mol Physiol.* 287(5):L928–L935.
23. Stryer L, Haugland RP (1967). Energy transfer: A spectroscopic ruler. *Proc Natl Acad Sci USA.* 58(2):719–726.
24. Rickert-Zacharias V, Schultz M, Mall MA, Schultz C (2021). Visualization of ectopic serine protease activity by förster resonance energy transfer-based reporters. *ACS Chem Biol.* 16(11):2174–2184.
25. Garty H, Palmer LG (1997). Epithelial sodium channels: Function, structure, and regulation. *Physiol Rev.* 77(2):359–396.
26. Bruns JB, Carattino MD, Sheng S, Maarouf AB, Weisz OA, Pilewski JM, Hughey RP, Kleyman TR (2007). Epithelial Na+ channels are fully activated by furin- and prostasin-dependent release of an inhibitory peptide from the gamma-subunit. *J Biol Chem.* 282(9):6153–6160.
27. Carattino MD, Mueller GM, Palmer LG, Frindt G, Rued AC, Hughey RP, Kleyman TR (2014). Prostasin interacts with the epithelial Na+ channel and facilitates cleavage of the γ-subunit by a second protease. *Am J Physiol Renal Physiol.* 307(9):F1080–F1087.
28. Zachar RM, Skjødt K, Marcussen N, Walter S, Toft A, Nielsen MR, Jensen BL, Svenningsen P (2015). The epithelial sodium channel

γ-subunit is processed proteolytically in human kidney. *J Am Soc Nephrol.* 26(1):95–106.

29. Tarran R, Button B, Picher M, Paradiso AM, Ribeiro CM, Lazarowski ER, Zhang L, Collins PL, Pickles RJ, Fredberg JJ, Boucher RC (2005). Normal and cystic fibrosis airway surface liquid homeostasis. The effects of phasic shear stress and viral infections. *J Biol Chem.* 280(42):35751–35759.

30. Livraghi-Butrico A, Wilkinson KJ, Volmer AS, Gilmore RC, Rogers TD, Caldwell RA, Burns KA, Esther CR Jr, Mall MA, Boucher RC, O'Neal WK, Grubb BR (2018). Lung disease phenotypes caused by over-expression of combinations of α-, β-, and γ-subunits of the epithelial sodium channel in mouse airways. *Am J Physiol Lung Cell Mol Physiol.* 314(2):L318–L331.

31. Verghese GM, Gutknecht MF, Caughey GH (2006). Prostasin regulates epithelial monolayer function: Cell-specific Gpld1-mediated secretion and functional role for GPI anchor. *Am J Physiol Cell Physiol.* 291(6):C1258–C1270.

Chapter 9

Prostasin in the Intestinal Tract

The intestinal epithelial cells are exposed to the stimuli and challenges from food, bacteria, and metabolites, and to other foreign insults constantly, and are renewed frequently to maintain the normal epithelial function. The cells at the crypt base proliferate and differentiate along the way up to the villus and are then removed into the lumen. This process takes about 3–4 days. The secretory progenitor cells differentiate into the tuft, goblet, Paneth, or enteroendocrine cells, and the absorptive progenitors differentiate into the enterocytes or M cells (Figure 9-1).

The colon constitutes the largest portion of the large intestine in the gastrointestinal tract and plays important roles in electrolyte and water absorption while maintaining and moving solid wastes along the tract. The epithelium covering the internal lumen side of the colon is formed with simple columnar epithelial cells. In addition to maintaining the body fluid homeostasis, this single columnar epithelial cell layer is also a major component of the intestinal mucosal barrier which is a heterogeneous fence separating the lumen of the colon from the body.

The epithelial cell self-renewal is an important process in the maintenance of tissue homeostasis. If the signaling molecules and networks that drive the differentiation process are interrupted, the intestinal cell functions cannot be maintained. Dysfunction of the intestinal mucosal barrier may be an early etiological event of many diseases such as the inflammatory bowel disease (IBD).

A properly differentiated, polarized, and tightly sealed epithelium is maintained by cell-cell junctions formed by cellular structural components. As illustrated below (Figure 9-2), the tight junctions (TJs)

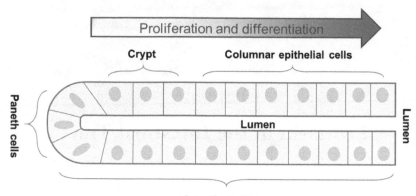

Figure 9-1. Schematic drawing of an intestinal villus. The arrow indicates the direction of the columnar epithelial cell proliferation and differentiation.

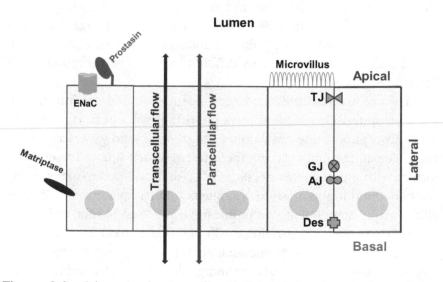

Figure 9-2. Schematic drawing of epithelial cell junctions and membrane compartment topology.

between the neighboring cells are formed near the apical/lumen side of the epithelium, the gap junctions (GJs) and the adherens junctions (AJs) are mostly formed at the basolateral side, while the desmosomes (Des) are at the basal side of the epithelial cells. AJs are mostly regulated by cadherins,

TJs are mostly regulated by claudins, occludins, ZO-1, and junctional adhesion molecules (JAMs)[1].

These junctions control the paracellular permeability of the colon epithelium while specific transporters and channels, such as the ENaC on the plasma membrane of the epithelial cells, control the transcellular permeability.

9.1 Prostasin regulates the colon epithelial permeability via matriptase

Prostasin is expressed in the colon and localized in the colon epithelial cells on the apical side. As a GPI-anchored serine protease, the entire prostasin polypeptide is positioned extracellularly to the lumen side of the epithelial cells. This unique cellular localization allows prostasin to interact with and work on other molecular and chemical entities in the intestinal lumen or co-localized on the membrane in the vicinity. The precise function of prostasin in the colon is unknown, but *in vitro* studies suggested that prostasin regulates the intestinal epithelial barrier closure in coordination with another membrane-anchored serine protease, matriptase[2]. Matriptase is a type-II transmembrane protein with a molecular mass of 95 kDa[3,4]. In polarized Caco2 human colon adenocarcinoma cells, matriptase is localized at the basolateral plasma membrane, away from the prostasin localization. It was suggested that for a transient interaction, a small fraction of the basolateral localized prostasin could activate matriptase[5]. The activated matriptase is subsequently involved in the barrier closure, establishing and maintaining a Caco2 cell layer impermeable to macromolecules such as the 4-kDa dextran, a commonly used tracer for testing the paracellular flux integrity. A leaky epithelium would allow a free passage of the dextran across through the epithelium from the apical to the basal side via the space in between the cells.

Interestingly, in mouse models where the prostasin gene (*Prss8*) is genetically and specifically silenced from expression in the colon epithelial cells, the permeability of the colonic epithelium is not compromised under normal living conditions. However, when challenged with dextran sodium sulfate (DSS), a chemical that induces colitis, the mouse colon mucosa presented a profound inflammation, with increased inflammatory cell infiltrations in the colon without prostasin expression, when compared to the mucosa with a normal colon prostasin expression[6,7]. The interaction of prostasin and matriptase in a complex environment *in vivo* may be different from what is seen *in vitro*, as there might be compensatory pathways that keep the colon epithelium permeability intact should prostasin function be comprised or diminished.

9.2 Prostasin regulates the colon electrolyte transport via the ENaC

The gastrointestinal tract is a major site of regulation of the body fluid homeostasis and is characterized as an aldosterone target tissue with differential expression of aldosterone receptors. Aldosterone enhances the expression of both the ENaC and the Na-K ATPase and promotes Na+ absorption from the apical/lumen side via the ENaC into the cell and Na+ export out of the cell into the body via the Na-K ATPase. The ENaC-mediated sodium transport across the cell is the rate-limiting step of epithelial sodium transport.

Aldosterone promotes electrogenic sodium reabsorption through the amiloride-sensitive ENaC by enhancing the insertion of ENaC subunits into the cell surface. When the Sprague-Dawley rats are fed with a zero-sodium diet for four weeks to induce aldosterone production or are infused with aldosterone continuously via an implanted osmotic pump for four weeks to mimic hyperaldosteronism, the prostasin mRNA expression is up-regulated in the distal colonic epithelial cells, which are sensitive to aldosterone regulation[8]. The increased prostasin could subsequently increase the open probability of the ENaC located on the apical cell membrane, providing an additional regulation of the sodium transport. These data suggested a possible prostasin regulation on the ENaC activity *in vivo* in the rat colon.

Perhaps the most telling demonstration that prostasin regulates the ENaC *in vivo* in the colon, was the study carried out by Malsure and colleagues[6] in 2014 in a transgenic mouse model. In this mouse model, the prostasin gene was knocked out in the intestinal epithelial cells by crossing the *Villin::Cre* transgenic mice that carry one *Prss8* allele and one *Prss8* knockout (D) allele[9] with the homozygous *Prss8*^lox/lox^ mice. The Cre recombinase expression was under the control of the mouse Villin 1 (*Vill* gene) promoter. The Cre recombinase mediates the loxP recombination of the loxP-flanked prostasin gene in the *Prss8*^lox/Δ^ mice. This resulted in a homozygous deletion of the prostasin gene in the villus and the crypt epithelial cells of the small and large intestines, a pattern that closely resembles that of the endogenous mouse *Vill* gene expression.

Overall, mice with the colon-specific deletion of the prostasin gene have no significant abnormalities at weaning, in terms of the Mendelian distribution of offspring, the whole-body weight of mice, food and water intake, urine or feces output, plasma and urinary sodium and potassium levels, the colon histology based on the number of crypt cells, the intestine length-to-body weight ratio, the intestinal permeability to dextran, and the expression levels of the ENaC subunits. However, the amiloride-sensitive rectal potential difference (ΔPD_{amil}) was significantly reduced in the prostasin knockout mice fed with the regular or a low-salt diet. In addition, the sodium content in the feces was high, even though the plasma aldosterone level was increased in the animals fed with the low-salt diet. In conclusion, the lack of prostasin expression in the mouse colon epithelial cells resulted in a reduced ENaC-mediated sodium transport from the colon lumen to the body, with an increased fecal sodium loss, even when the dietary salt was limited.

Interestingly, the lack of prostasin expression in the colon epithelial cells did not impair the barrier function, as the permeability of the colon epithelium was unaffected. This result was contrary to that reported for mice lacking prostasin in the skin, in which a severely impaired epidermal barrier was documented[9]. The cause of this discrepancy is unclear. Another interesting finding in this study was that the ENaC subunits detected in the mouse colon epithelial cells had both the full-length and the cleaved forms in a western blot analysis, suggesting that the regulation of the ENaC activity is not solely dependent on the prostasin proteolytic cleavage of the ENaC subunits. This observation is consistent with the findings in the lung of a prostasin knockout model[10].

However, in the kidney, it was suggested that prostasin is responsible for the final activation of the ENaC subunits by a proteolytic cleavage to remove the inhibitory peptide from the γ-subunit[11].

9.3 Prostasin regulates the intestinal epithelium integrity via SPINT2

Autosomal recessive congenital tufting enteropathy (CTE) and congenital sodium diarrhea (CSD) are rare disorders characterized mainly by a watery and high sodium diarrhea after birth and during infancy. The high fecal sodium loss often leads to an electrolyte imbalance and dehydration, a life-threatening condition in the first few months of life. Genetic alterations responsible for these disorders are believed to be a mutated *EPCAM* gene (2p21) in 73% of the non-syndromic CTE patients or a mutated *SPINT2* gene (19q13.2) in 21% of the syndromic CSD patients. The histological phenotype of the intestinal epithelium presents with villous atrophy, crypt hyperplasia, focal epithelial tufts, and ill-developed and ill-differentiated enterocytes in the CTE patients, while only a mild to moderate intestinal villus atrophy is observed in the CSD patients. Enterocytes are intestinal absorptive and simple columnar epithelial cells that line the inner surface of the small and large intestines. They are responsible for taking up small molecules and nutrients from the intestinal lumen. Microvilli increase the apical surface of the lining for molecular transports.

An epithelial cell adhesion molecule (EpCAM) mutation was identified as the primary cause for CTE in a family, by using the Affymetrix 50K single nucleotide polymorphism (SNP) chips[12]. The EpCAM is localized to the cell-cell junctions and regulates the junction formation in the intestinal epithelium by recruiting and forming a complex with the claudin-7 protein, a key component of the tight junction of the enterocytes. Destabilization of the EpCAM-claudin-7 complex compromises the tight junction architecture, leading to a leaky gastrointestinal (GI) epithelium, which is the molecular basis of the watery diarrhea and sodium loss.

Mutations in the gene encoding the Kunitz-type serine protease inhibitor 2 were reported in a syndromic form of CSD based on a genomic-wide SNP scan, associated with the gene mutations is a loss-of-function of the protein SPINT2 encoded by *SPINT2*[13].

SPINT2, aka, hepatocyte growth factor activator inhibitor-2 (HAI-2) is indispensable in normal physiology, especially in tissues/organs where HAI-2 expression is high, such as the intestinal tract. In a mouse model, a specific ablation of the *Sprint2* gene in adult mouse intestines for six days resulted in death[14]. In fact, within three days of the ablation, the GI tract began to shrink in length, the mucosal barriers were dissolving, and the villi appeared atrophic. These phenotypes resemble the clinical manifestations of the CTE patients. In addition, lacking the HAI-2 protein in the enterocytes impaired the enterocyte differentiation and the architecture of the GI epithelium. At the molecular level, an insufficient HAI-2 presence in the epithelium correlated with a lesser EpCAM protein expression on the cell surface and a lesser claudin-7 protein expression. At the histological level, an acute inactivation of HAI-2 in mouse intestinal epithelial cells induced epithelial cell apoptosis and a compensatory proliferation. However, due to the abnormal proliferation, the organization of the tissue was affected, manifested by the exfoliation of the mucosa, atrophic villi, tufts formation of enterocytes, and elongated crypts. These histological changes resemble the syndromic form of CSD.

Indeed, in 2019, Holt-Danborg and colleagues[15] identified HAI-2 mutations in patients with the syndromic form of congenital sodium diarrhea (SCSD). A reduced inhibitory activity of the mutated HAI-2 towards prostasin, but not matriptase, was noted. The molecular mechanism was ascertained by a structural model of the KD2 domain of the human HAI-2 using the protein structure predication software I-TASSER. Mutations in the KD2 domain at Phe161, Tyr163, or Gly168 affected KD2 folding and the access by prostasin. The authors suggested that KD2 may be the exosite for prostasin-KD1 interaction, but not required for matriptase-KD1 binding.

It has been hypothesized, investigated, and reported in many studies that in the intestinal epithelial cells, the EpCAM stabilizes claudin-7 by forming a complex during tight junction formation. Matriptase could cleave the EpCAM and dissociate it from claudin-7[16]. A loss of HAI-2 inhibition leads to matriptase over-activation and an increased cleavage of the EpCAM[17]. Currently, a modified hypothesis is formulated in which prostasin, a matriptase-cutting and -activating enzyme, is tightly controlled by HAI-2 in the intestinal epithelial cells[18], as the activated prostasin in a complex with HAI-2 is detected in the human intestine tissue and the Caco-2 cells[19]. A reduced or absent HAI-2 inhibition results in a constitutive activation of prostasin, a condition that triggers a functionally linked chain of events starting with an over-activation of matriptase, followed by EpCAM cleavage, claudin-7 destabilization from the tight junctions, and an increased mucosal permeability. Indeed, in an organoid crypt culture silencing the prostasin expression can rescue the organoid failure caused by the *Spint2* ablation[14]. Further, a deletion of the HAI-2 gene in mice is embryonic lethal, but not if the deletion of the HAI-2 is accompanied with a reduced prostasin activity[20], as observed in a double transgenic mouse model of *Spint2$^{-/-}$;Prss8$^{R44Q/R44Q}$*. The R44Q prostasin variant is resistant to the proteolytic activation, but itself is biologically active[21]. However, the *Spint2$^{-/-}$;Prss8$^{R44Q/R44Q}$* transgenic mice do not survive over a week after birth. A possible reason could be that the functional prostasin present in the nursing mother's milk triggers the matriptase activation in the pups' GI tract due to the lack of HAI-2 inhibition.

Finally, a prostasin over-activation could cause an ENaC over-activation and the subsequent high Na$^+$ and water intake by the colon epithelial cells, with less Na$^+$ and water in the feces. A loss/reduction of function due to SPINT2 mutations leaves the prostasin activity under-inhibited and leads to an increased matriptase activation and a subsequent colon epithelial junction dissolution, with Na$^+$ and water loss in the feces. Two different outcomes can be mechanistically associated with prostasin over-activation and seem to be contradicting to each other. This, however, reflects exactly the multifaceted functional presence of prostasin in the colon epithelium with the requirements of maintaining its tissue architecture and performing the diverse and sophisticated functions. Prostasin's role in one aspect of the colon epithelial function may seem to have an adverse effect on another aspect. It is perhaps the very reason that an active prostasin serine protease in an epithelial tissue cannot be absent but also cannot be in great excess. This hypothesis was supported in an *in vitro* trophoblast cell line study, in which the phenotype of an impaired transepithelial resistance is the same in cells with an over-expression of prostasin or with the prostasin expression silenced[22]. The regulation of prostasin action requires specific molecular mechanisms as well as cellular compartmentation, and even differential timing with regard to when, where, and how much prostasin is needed and allowed. Presumably the impact of prostasin on ENaC activation is only relevant with the proper formation of the epithelium, wherein its impact on matriptase and EpCAM is ahead in the timing of a development course, during the epithelial maturation. In an adult animal, the prostasin→matriptase→junction dissolution pathway following the HAI-2 loss is the dominant outcome, as the structural damage is so massive that the sodium and water transport function through prostasin→ENaC becomes moot.

A great deal of knowledge and information have been gained on prostasin since its discovery a short 30 years ago. Much of the gain was and could only have been made with studies using either *in vitro* cell culture systems or animal models, involving an over-expression or an expression silencing of prostasin, or a takeaway of a prostasin inhibitor or an over-supply of the inhibitor. These studies can provide a clue and a picture of what prostasin's function may be in a specific aspect of the overall tissue and organ function, but the when, where, and how much in the biological context are important in the interpretation and reconciliation of the results. An experimental genetic manipulation is fixed and the outcome permanent, but in the organ and tissue of a living person, the activity of prostasin may very well be under the control of transient mechanisms. These may involve reversible epigenetic modifications of DNA and the chromatin to affect the expression, especially in a tissue with a renewal agenda like the colon and food-borne factors that impact the protease activity.

Returning to the opening remarks on the physiological functions of the colon, a major one is the Na^+ and water balance, and movement of the solid waste. The colon is also the residence of the intestinal flora of microbes, which can have a major impact on the functions of the colon with far reaching health or disease impacts. Fecal transplant therapy is proving to be effective in modulating the therapeutic efficacy of monoclonal antibodies targeting the immune checkpoint for cancer treatment, eliciting a response in non-responding patients receiving the fecal transplant from the responders. There is currently no reported research outcome on how the changes in the gut flora would affect the expression and function of prostasin, or vice versa. There has been some limited research on the impact of matriptase deficiency to the skin microbiome[23]. It would not be a wild suggestion, given the regulating role of prostasin in innate immunity, that it may have an impact on the gut microbiome-host interaction. Prostasin's role in innate immunity will be detailed in a later chapter.

References

1. Tsukita S, Furuse M, Itoh M (2001). Multifunctional strands in tight junctions. *Nat Rev Mol Cell Biol*. 2(4):285–293.
2. Buzza MS, Martin EW, Driesbaugh KH, Désilets A, Leduc R, Antalis TM (2013). Prostasin is required for matriptase activation in intestinal epithelial cells to regulate closure of the paracellular pathway. *J Biol Chem*. 288(15):10328–10337.
3. Lin CY, Anders J, Johnson M, Sang QA, Dickson RB (1999). Molecular cloning of cDNA for matriptase, a matrix-degrading serine protease with trypsin-like activity. *J Biol Chem*. 274(26):18231–18236.
4. Takeuchi T, Shuman MA, Craik CS (1999). Reverse biochemistry: Use of macromolecular protease inhibitors to dissect complex biological processes and identify a membrane-type serine protease in epithelial cancer and normal tissue. *Proc Natl Acad Sci USA*. 96(20):11054–11061.
5. Friis S, Godiksen S, Bornholdt J, Selzer-Plon J, Rasmussen HB, Bugge TH, Lin CY, Vogel LK (2011). Transport via the transcytotic pathway makes prostasin available as a substrate for matriptase. *J Biol Chem*. 286(7):5793–5802.
6. Malsure S, Wang Q, Charles RP, Sergi C, Perrier R, Christensen BM, Maillard M, Rossier BC, Hummler E (2014). Colon-specific deletion of epithelial sodium channel causes sodium loss and aldosterone resistance. *J Am Soc Nephrol*. 25(7):1453–1464.
7. Sugitani Y, Nishida A, Inatomi O, Ohno M, Imai T, Kawahara M, Kitamura K, Andoh A (2020). Sodium absorption stimulator prostasin (PRSS8) has an anti-inflammatory effect via downregulation of TLR4 signaling in inflammatory bowel disease. *J Gastroenterol*. 55(4):408–417.

8. Fukushima K, Naito H, Funayama Y, Yonezawa H, Haneda S, Shibata C, Sasaki I (2004). In vivo induction of prostasin mRNA in colonic epithelial cells by dietary sodium depletion and aldosterone infusion in rats. *J Gastroenterol.* 39(10):940–947.

9. Leyvraz C, Charles RP, Rubera I, Guitard M, Rotman S, Breiden B, Sandhoff K, Hummler E (2005). The epidermal barrier function is dependent on the serine protease CAP1/Prss8. *J Cell Biol.* 170(3):487–496.

10. Planès C, Randrianarison NH, Charles RP, Frateschi S, Cluzeaud F, Vuagniaux G, Soler P, Clerici C, Rossier BC, Hummler E (2010). ENaC-mediated alveolar fluid clearance and lung fluid balance depend on the channel-activating protease 1. *EMBO Mol Med.* 2(1):26–37.

11. Bruns JB, Carattino MD, Sheng S, Maarouf AB, Weisz OA, Pilewski JM, Hughey RP, Kleyman TR (2007). Epithelial Na+ channels are fully activated by furin- and prostasin-dependent release of an inhibitory peptide from the gamma-subunit. *J Biol Chem.* 282(9):6153–6160.

12. Sivagnanam M, Mueller JL, Lee H, Chen Z, Nelson SF, Turner D, Zlotkin SH, Pencharz PB, Ngan BY, Libiger O, Schork NJ, Lavine JE, Taylor S, Newbury RO, Kolodner RD, Hoffman HM (2008). Identification of EpCAM as the gene for congenital tufting enteropathy. *Gastroenterology.* 135(2):429–437.

13. Heinz-Erian P, Müller T, Krabichler B, Schranz M, Becker C, Rüschendorf F, Nürnberg P, Rossier B, Vujic M, Booth IW, Holmberg C, Wijmenga C, Grigelioniene G, Kneepkens CMF, Rosipal S, Mistrik M, Kappler M, Michaud L, Dóczy LC, Siu VM, Krantz M, Zoller H, Utermann G, Janecke AR (2009). Mutations in SPINT2 cause a syndromic form of congenital sodium diarrhea. *Am J Hum Genet.* 84(2):188–196.

14. Kawaguchi M, Yamamoto K, Takeda N, Fukushima T, Yamashita F, Sato K, Kitamura K, Hippo Y, Janetka JW, Kataoka H (2019). Hepatocyte growth factor activator inhibitor-2 stabilizes Epcam and maintains epithelial organization in the mouse intestine. *Commun Biol.* 2:11.

15. Holt-Danborg L, Vodopiutz J, Nonboe AW, De Laffolie J, Skovbjerg S, Wolters VM, Müller T, Hetzer B, Querfurt A, Zimmer KP, Jensen JK, Entenmann A, Heinz-Erian P, Vogel LK, Janecke AR (2019). SPINT2 (HAI-2) missense variants identified in congenital sodium diarrhea/tufting enteropathy affect the ability of HAI-2 to inhibit prostasin but not matriptase. *Hum Mol Genet.* 28(5):828–841.

16. Wu CJ, Feng X, Lu M, Morimura S, Udey MC (2017). Matriptase-mediated cleavage of EpCAM destabilizes claudins and dysregulates intestinal epithelial homeostasis. *J Clin Invest.* 127(2):623–634.

17. Szabo R, Callies LK, Bugge TH (2019). Matriptase drives early-onset intestinal failure in a mouse model of congenital tufting enteropathy. *Development*. 146(22):dev183392.

18. Shiao F, Liu LO, Huang N, Lai YJ, Barndt RJ, Tseng CC, Wang JK, Jia B, Johnson MD, Lin CY (2017). Selective inhibition of prostasin in human enterocytes by the integral membrane kunitz-type serine protease inhibitor HAI-2. *PLoS One*. 12(1):e0170944.

19. Barndt RB, Lee MJ, Huang N, Lu DD, Lee SC, Du PW, Chang CC, Tsai PB, Huang YK, Chang HM, Wang JK, Lai CH, Johnson MD, Lin CY (2021). Targeted HAI-2 deletion causes excessive proteolysis with pro-longed active prostasin and depletion of HAI-1 monomer in intestinal but not epidermal epithelial cells. *Hum Mol Genet*. 30(19):1833–1850.

20. Szabo R, Bugge TH (2018). Loss of HAI-2 in mice with decreased pros-tasin activity leads to an early-onset intestinal failure resembling congeni-tal tufting enteropathy. *PLoS One*. 13(4):e0194660.

21. Friis S, Uzzun Sales K, Godiksen S, Peters DE, Lin CY, Vogel LK, Bugge TH (2013). A matriptase-prostasin reciprocal zymogen activation com-plex with unique features: Prostasin as a non-enzymatic co-factor for matriptase activation. *J Biol Chem*. 288(26):19028–19039.

22. Chai AC, Robinson AL, Chai KX, Chen LM (2015). Ibuprofen regulates the expression and function of membrane-associated serine proteases prostasin and matriptase. *BMC Cancer*. 15:1025.

23. Scharschmidt TC, List K, Grice EA, Szabo R, NISC Comparative Sequencing Program, Renaud G, Lee CC, Wolfsberg TG, Bugge TH, Segre JA (2009). Matriptase-deficient mice exhibit ichthyotic skin with a selective shift in skin microbiota. *J Invest Dermatol*. 129(10):2435–2442.

Chapter 10

Prostasin in the Skin

The skin is the largest organ of a human body and has many important functions. As a physical barrier, the skin protects the body from the insults of microorganisms in the environment and the ultraviolet radiation from the sunlight. More important, the skin as an organ maintains the body's water and electrolyte homeostasis, serves as sensors for pain during injuries and for the change of temperature and humidity in the surroundings, and functions as the sentinel in innate immunity.

The human skin is composed of three layers, from the outermost, the epidermis, the dermis, and the hypodermis. The dermis is rich in collagen and elastin, making up 90% of the skin thickness, with hair follicles, nerves, sweat glands, and blood vessels. The hypodermis is a fatty layer with connective tissues to muscles and bones, regulating the body temperature. The outermost epidermis layer contains viable keratinocytes.

Keratinocytes are epithelial cells, among them some are capable of self-renewing throughout the adult life, being the functional unit of epidermal proliferation. There are 4–5 cell layers of keratinocytes stacked in the epidermis. As they move upwards from the basal proliferating layer to the outermost maturing layer, keratinocytes lose their proliferating ability and undergo differentiation and enucleation, and finally become the anucleated corneocytes, which are the principal cells of the stratum corneum layer (Figure 10-1).

In the granular layer, keratinocytes produce the filamentous keratin proteins which interact with filaggrin to form a keratin-filaggrin-based protein matrix and the aggregated fibers. These structures are the

111

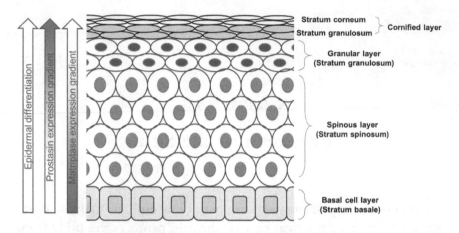

Figure 10-1. Schematic drawing of the skin epidermis layers. Arrows show the direction of the events. The darker blue color in the arrows represents a higher expression level of the protein.

main component and the foundation of the envelope of corneocytes entering the stratum corneum layer. Filaggrins are histidine-rich and highly basic proteins derived from their precursor proteins called pro-filaggrins (>400 kDa) expressed in the granular layer. Upon proteolytic cleavage by proteases, profilaggrins are dephosphorylated and become the smaller and functional filaggrin monomers (~40 kDa) during the maturation of keratinocytes from the granular layer to the corneocyte layer. When the corneocytes are moving to the further uppermost layers of the stratum corneum, filaggrin is further degraded into free amino acids which are hydroscopic molecules capable of holding water and therefore are referred to as the natural moisturizing factor (NMF). The degradation of filaggrin occurs only when the corneocytes are mature and located at the superficial layers of the stratum corneum. The NMF plays major parts in the hydration, barrier homeostasis, desquamation, and plasticity of the skin. An appropriate stratum corneum hydration, especially with the NMF-bound water, is essential to protecting the skin from dehydration.

The functional significance of filaggrin generation and degradation is illustrated with the loss-of-function mutations in the filaggrin gene (*FLG*). Several skin diseases have been attributed to improper functions of filaggrin, such as ichthyosis vulgaris and atopic dermatitis (AD). The patients have significantly lower levels of the NMF in the stratum corneum and a high transepidermal water loss.

Lipid molecules are synthesized in the upper spinous layer, accumulating in the granular layer and released to the extracellular spaces between the granular layer and the cornified layer[1]. Transglutaminases mediate the crosslinking of the cornified envelope proteins and the linkage with the extracellular lipids to form an impermeable skin surface. Crosslinking also happens between adhesion proteins in the desmosomal complexes in the upper granular layer. Other intercellular adhesions including the adherens junctions and the tight junctions are also instrumental to the formation and the integrity of the epidermal barrier. The cell-cell junctional proteins claudins and occludins are the main components of the tight junction, which is critical in the regulation of paracellular transport of water and solutes as well as the permeability of the epidermal layers.

The protective barrier function of the skin develops during the period between Week 20 of gestation to birth. The number of cell layers increases in the epidermis and the dermal-epidermal junction forms. The infant skin, by comparison to the adult skin, has a weaker barrier function as indicated by an increased trans-epidermal water loss (TEWL)[2] and a lower water-holding capacity[3], and has a higher epidermal proliferation rate[4]. The skin continues to mature after birth and the surface of the skin refreshes itself continuously. Keratinocytes proliferate at the basal layer of the epidermis and migrate outwards toward the skin surface while differentiating and gaining the barrier function. As an impermeable seal for the skin, the outermost layer of the epidermis, the stratum corneum, sheds off and refreshes every 7–8 weeks, a process referred to as desquamation.

The time of birth marks a significant change for the lung alveolar cells as they experience a fast transition from a fluid-filled environment to a gaseous environment, this is also true for the skin. Before birth, the skin is soaked in the amniotic fluid but transits to the air environment after birth. The difference is that the lung fluid needs to be removed to allow for air exposure, and this removal is accomplished partially by the coordinated actions of prostasin and the ENaC. For the skin however, the change from inside the amniotic-fluid-filled sac to outside in the air imposes an immediate need to protect against water loss. To adapt to this transition, the neonatal skin reduces its permeability to retain water inside the skin.

Prostasin participates in establishing and maintaining the tight junction integrity and regulating the paracellular permeability in various epithelia. Unlike in the lung or kidney epithelium, prostasin is not a critical regulator of the skin ENaC activity because the skin ENaC is functional when the prostasin gene is knocked out in the skin. Rather, prostasin regulates the skin tight junction to prevent excessive body fluid loss, keeping the skin in the hydrated state.

In 2005, Leyvraz and colleagues[5] reported that mice with a targeted deletion of the prostasin gene in the epidermis die within 60 hours after birth. The stratum corneum in these mice is severely malformed with an abnormal lipid composition, enlarged corneocytes, improper filaggrin processing, and ill-organized occludin proteins in the tight junction. The sealing of the skin is compromised, the permeability is high, and the body weight is quickly lost due to the loss of water within hours after birth. Essentially, the pups die from a severe dehydration. In the following year, Netzel-Arnette and colleagues[6] suggested that matriptase is the upstream enzyme responsible for prostasin activation in the mouse skin by cleaving the latter into two chains. The hypothesis was based on the co-localization of the two proteases in the epidermis of mice and the presence of the two-chain prostasin protein in the mouse epidermis lysate but not in that of the matriptase-deficient mice.

In 2016, Lai and colleagues[7] reported that both prostasin and matriptase are expressed in the human skin but mostly residing in different sublayers of the epidermis. Prostasin is detected primarily in differentiated cells in the granular layer and activated[8], while matriptase is mainly located in basal keratinocytes. There is some co-localization of prostasin and matriptase seen in the keratinocytes transitioning from the proliferation state to the differentiation state, but the two proteins are localized in different compartments in the same keratinocyte. Prostasin is seen as polarized patches in the cell while matriptase is localized at the intercellular junctions. A similar pattern of such discrete localization of prostasin and matriptase in the human skin was confirmed later by Liao and colleagues[9] in 2022. It appears that prostasin and matriptase could not activate each other in the human skin as the two proteins are localized in different cellular compartments in a keratinocyte and in differential layers of the epidermis.

In 2020, Chang and colleagues[10] performed a series of experiments comparing the prostasin and matriptase expression and function in the epidermis during injury and in the normal quiescent state. They reported that in the human skin, prostasin is expressed at the highest level in the uppermost layers of the viable cells, and the expression level is increased during the skin injury and recovery periods, while matriptase is mostly expressed in the periphery of the basal and spinous keratinocytes. The co-localization of prostasin and matriptase proteins is minimal in cells in the epidermis. This contrasts with the observations made in the mouse skin where prostasin and matriptase are co-localized. In addition, prostasin seems to be constitutively activated in unidentified organelle-like structures of the granular keratinocytes, but matriptase is predominantly in the zymogen form in the basal and spinous keratinocytes.

It may be possible that prostasin is required and activated for keratinocyte differentiation during the maturation process. Whereas, matriptase may play roles more in keratinocyte proliferation than in the differentiation[11]. The prostasin zymogen may be activated by matriptase in the lower layer of the epidermis, e.g., the granular keratinocytes. Along the way of moving upwards during keratinocyte maturation, the activated prostasin could trigger matriptase activation and auto-activation, and eliminate matriptase from the fully mature cells.

The type-II transmembrane extracellular serine protease matriptase is synthesized as a zymogen but upon activation, mediates its own shedding from the plasma membrane via a *de novo* proteolytic cleavage at Arg186 between the SEA (Sperm protein, Enterokinase and Agrin) domain and the CUB (complement C1r/C1s, Uegf, Bmp1) domain in its extracellular domain (ECD)[12]. The shed-off matriptase is the bulk of its ECD including the carboxyl-terminal protease domain, implicated for proteolytic functional roles in the extracellular environment. The shedding leaves behind only the SEA domain, reducing or eliminating signals in an immunohistochemical examination for its expression in tissues.

The half-life of prostasin is long, so the positive staining of prostasin protein in the uppermost outer layer of the skin is a reflection of the accumulated and activated prostasin serving functions in maintaining the tight junction structure and the hydration state. On one hand, there may be no mechanism to remove prostasin in the anucleated corneocytes, except through shedding off during desquamation. On the other hand, matriptase may need to be removed in the mature keratinocytes, especially in the anucleated corneocytes. For this, once prostasin is activated by matriptase when keratinocytes enter into the late differentiation phase, the active prostasin activates the matriptase zymogen to initiate a matriptase auto-activation cascade, removing matriptase from the cells. The activated matriptase is complexed with HAI-1 for inactivation and removal from the cells. HAI-1 is reported to be the main inhibitor for both matriptase and prostasin in the skin, but not HAI-2[13–15].

In summary, keratinocytes proliferate in the basal layer, gradually transit and mature while moving upward through the spinous layer and the granulosa layer, ending in the corneum layer. Each layer is defined by how mature the keratinocytes are in that layer or what functions the keratinocyte can perform therein. The entire process is quite dynamic. The same keratinocyte at different maturation states can perform the proper physiological functions by stage. For example, matriptase is involved in keratinocyte proliferation and it is predominantly expressed and localized in the basal layer. Prostasin is responsible for keratinocyte differentiation and may be activated in the basal spinous layer or the granular layer by matriptase when maturation begins, as the activated prostasin can be seen in those layers. The activated prostasin will quickly initiate matriptase zymogen activation and auto-activation of additional zymogens, and then matriptase is eliminated from the maturing keratinocytes. Meanwhile the activated prostasin is retained in the maturing keratinocytes and plays roles in the final differentiation of keratinocytes. Until the keratinocyte is fully mature and becomes the enucleated corneocyte, prostasin is required in the whole differentiation process. Even in the stratum corneum layer in which no viable cells are present but only dead cornified cells, prostasin may still be required for barrier function as the stratum corneum is recognized as being biochemically active although biologically dead[16].

Only when maturation takes place, keratin and filaggrin start to interact with each other to form the matrix and keep the corneocytes in the flat shape. Filaggrin degradation to free amino acids happens in the stratum corneum where the NMF builds up, and the skin hydration status affects this degradation process. Therefore, prostasin is essential in skin epidermal differentiation. An absence of prostasin in the skin produces an undifferentiated epidermis with functional defects, unable to form a proper barrier when the skin is exposed to the dry air after the transition from the amniotic fluid state, as seen in the prostasin knockout mouse model. If the matriptase activity is not controlled and the matriptase protein is not removed near the end of keratinocyte maturation, excess matriptase may compromise the integrity of the skin and diseases may form, such as ichthyosis vulgaris and atopic dermatitis. In this sense, perhaps one of the functions of prostasin is to limit the matriptase presence and activity in the terminally differentiated epithelial cells.

References

1. Elias PM, Wakefield JS (2014). Mechanisms of abnormal lamellar body secretion and the dysfunctional skin barrier in patients with atopic dermatitis. *J Allergy Clin Immunol.* 134(4):781–791.e1.
2. Nikolovski J, Stamatas GN, Kollias N, Wiegand BC (2008). Barrier function and water-holding and transport properties of infant stratum corneum are different from adult and continue to develop through the first year of life. *J Invest Dermatol.* 128(7):1728–1736.
3. Saijo S and Tagami H (1991). Dry skin of newborn infants: Functional analysis of the stratum corneum. *Pediatr Dermatol.* 8(2):155–159.
4. Stamatas GN, Nikolovski J, Luedtke MA, Kollias N, Wiegand BC (2010). Infant skin microstructure assessed in vivo differs from adult skin in organization and at the cellular level. *Pediatr Dermatol.* 27(2):125–131.
5. Leyvraz C, Charles RP, Rubera I, Guitard M, Rotman S, Breiden B, Sandhoff K, Hummler E (2005). The epidermal barrier function is dependent on the serine protease CAP1/Prss8. *J Cell Biol.* 170(3):487–496.

6. Netzel-Arnett S, Currie BM, Szabo R, Lin CY, Chen LM, Chai KX, Antalis TM, Bugge TH, List K (2006). Evidence for a matriptase-prostasin proteolytic cascade regulating terminal epidermal differentiation. *J Biol Chem.* 281(44):32941–32945.

7. Lai CH, Chang SC, Chen YJ, Wang YJ, Lai YJ, Chang HD, Berens EB, Johnson MD, Wang JK, Lin CY (2016). Matriptase and prostasin are expressed in human skin in an inverse trend over the course of differentiation and are targeted to different regions of the plasma membrane. *Biol Open.* 5(10):1380–1387.

8. Lee SP, Kao CY, Chang SC, Chiu YL, Chen YJ, Chen MG, Chang CC, Lin YW, Chiang CP, Wang JK, Lin CY, Johnson MD (2018). Tissue distribution and subcellular localizations determine in vivo functional relationship among prostasin, matriptase, HAI-1, and HAI-2 in human skin. *PLoS One.* 13(2):e0192632.

9. Liao AH, Chen YC, Chen CY, Chang SC, Chuang HC, Lin DL, Chiang CP, Wang CH, Wang JK (2022). Mechanisms of ultrasound-microbubble cavitation for inducing the permeability of human skin. *J Control Release.* 349:388–400.

10. Chang SC, Chiang CP, Lai CH, Du PA, Hung YS, Chen YH, Yang HY, Fang HY, Lee SP, Tang HJ, Wang JK, Johnson MD, Lin CY (2020). Matriptase and prostasin proteolytic activities are differentially regulated in normal and wounded skin. *Hum Cell.* 33(4):990–1005.

11. Chen YW, Wang JK, Chou FP, Wu BY, Hsiao HC, Chiu H, Xu Z, Baksh ANH, Shi G, Kaul M, Barndt R, Shanmugam VK, Johnson MD, Lin CY (2014). Matriptase regulates proliferation and early, but not terminal, differentiation of human keratinocytes. *J Invest Dermatol.* 134(2):405–414.

12. Tseng CC, Jia B, Barndt R, Gu Y, Chen CY, Tseng IC, Su SF, Wang JK, Johnson MD, Lin CY (2017). Matriptase shedding is closely coupled with matriptase zymogen activation and requires de novo proteolytic cleavage likely involving its own activity. *PLoS One.* 12(8):e0183507.

13. Chen YW, Wang JK, Chou FP, Chen CY, Rorke EA, Chen LM, Chai KX, Eckert RL, Johnson MD, Lin CY (2010). Regulation of the matriptase-prostasin cell surface proteolytic cascade by hepatocyte growth factor activator inhibitor-1 during epidermal differentiation. *J Biol Chem.* 285(41):31755–31762.

14. Tseng IC, Xu H, Chou FP, Li G, Vazzano AP, Kao JP, Johnson MD, Lin CY (2010). Matriptase activation, an early cellular response to acidosis. *J Biol Chem.* 285(5):3261–3270.

15. Chu LL, Xu Y, Yang JR, Hu YA, Chang HH, Lai HY, Tseng CC, Wang HY, Johnson MD, Wang JK, Lin CY (2014). Human cancer cells retain modest levels of enzymatically active matriptase only in extracellular milieu following induction of zymogen activation. *PLoS One.* 9(3):e92244.

16. Richter T, Peuckert C, Sattler M, Koenig K, Riemann I, Hintze U, Wittern KP, Wiesendanger R, Wepf R (2004). Dead but highly dynamic — the stratum corneum is divided into three hydration zones. *Skin Pharmacol Physiol.* 17(5):246–257.

Chapter 11

Prostasin in the Reproductive Organs

The human prostasin was discovered and isolated from the seminal plasma as a serine protease with an affinity to the serine protease inhibitor aprotinin. It is present in the seminal plasma at a level of >8 µg/ml, which raises the question of whether prostasin would have a role in reproductive biology. The prostate-specific antigen (PSA/hK3), a serine protease of the tissue kallikrein family at a much higher level in the seminal plasma, averaging to several hundred micrograms per milliliter, has a role in proteolytic degradation of semenogelins and thus semen liquefaction and promotion of sperm motility. Unlike the PSA, a secreted protease, prostasin is membrane-anchored, but can be shed-off via the actions of phospholipases or exported in the lipid vesicles known as the exosomes, or specifically, prostasomes in the seminal plasma. This simple structural comparison would suggest for potentially different functional roles of prostasin than liquefaction as the competition from the PSA would be stiff and overwhelming.

The primary human reproductive organs are the ovaries and the testes. They produce the haploid gametes, i.e., the eggs and the sperm. The secondary reproductive organs include the fallopian tubes, the uterus, the vagina, the accessory glands, and the external genitalia in females; and the excretory ducts of the epididymis, the ductus deferens/vas deferens, the ejaculatory ducts, the seminal vesicles, the prostate, the bulbourethral glands, and the penis in males.

Human reproduction on the female side, begins when a dominant follicle develops to its maturity in the ovary, then releases the ovum outside the ovary. From there, the nearby fallopian tube captures the ovum, which may be fertilized by a sperm inside the fallopian tube, forming the zygote. The zygote begins to divide to form a cluster of cells called the blastocyst, which subsequently moves into the uterus, hatches from the zona pellucida, burrows into the endometrium, and implants into the uterine wall.

The blastocyst consists of a fluid-filled cavity, the inner cell mass of the embryoblast, and the outer cell mass of the trophoblast. The embryoblast, the initial structure of the embryo, is further differentiated into a bilaminar disc containing the hypoblast layer and the epiblast layer. The different layers of cells eventually differentiate into the various tissues and organs of the body. The trophoblast, the origin of the placenta, differentiates into the inner layer cytotrophoblast and the outer layer syncytiotrophoblast. The placenta is formed from the outer trophoblast layer. As the syncytiotrophoblast expands and forms the lacunae inside the endometrium, the endometrium capillaries are remodeled to form the maternal sinusoids and begin to connect with the lacunae to produce the lacunar networks, the foundation of the mature placenta capable of exchanging oxygen, nutrients, and metabolites between the fetus and the mother (Figure 11-1).

The process of embryo implantation is mediated by trophoblast invasion, a property that is reminiscent of malignant cancer cells. The trophoblast invasion is necessary for remodeling the maternal spiral arteries and establishing the uteroplacental circulation. The difference between the trophoblast cells and cancer cells is that the trophoblast

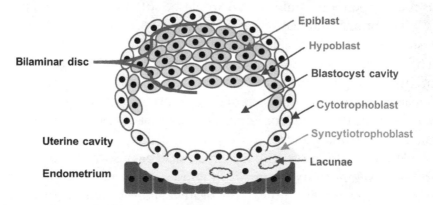

Figure 11-1.   The trophoblast and the embryoblast in a blastocyst.

invasion is under strict control to limit the invasion to the implantation site during a pregnancy. A proper trophoblast invasion determines the placental efficiency and fetal viability in the late gestation stages. Conversely, an inefficient trophoblast invasion could result in adverse pregnancy outcomes, e.g., intrauterine growth restriction (IUGR), or preeclampsia[1].

Serine proteases including the urokinase-type plasminogen activator (uPA) and the tissue-type plasminogen activator (tPA) are implicated in the formation of the placental villi, where they cleave plasminogen to generate plasmin, which is an extracellular matrix (ECM) degrading enzyme. Plasminogen activator inhibitor-1 (PAI-1) inhibits the uPA to limit the trophoblast invasion. It is this balance of activating and inhibiting forces on proteolysis, cell proliferation, and differentiation that governs the trophoblastic invasion to its perfection. It has been reported that transforming growth factor β (TGFβ) produced by the endometrial decidual cells is a major regulator in limiting the trophoblast invasion. TGFβ provides the signals to direct the invasive and proliferative trophoblast cells to become the non-invasive, fused, and multinucleated syncytiotrophoblasts at the fetal-maternal interface[2,3]. The syncytiotrophoblast (ST) is considered as an epithelial barrier covering the vascular placental villi, protecting the fetus from the maternal immune attack, but permitting the passage of nutrients and oxygen. Interestingly, TGFβ is also an inhibitor of prostasin gene expression *in vitro*[4].

In 2006, Lin and colleagues[5] investigated the prostasin expression in rhesus monkey (Macaca mulatta) endometrium and placenta during early pregnancy and showed that prostasin is expressed during embryo implantation at trophoblast invasion and formation of the placenta. Prostasin expression is initially localized in the uterine endometrium glandular epithelium on Day 12 and diminished progressively on Day 18 and Day 26 of pregnancy. During the same period, prostasin expression is increased progressively in the placental villi, the trophoblastic column, the trophoblastic shell, and the fetal-maternal border from Day 12 (lacunar stage) to Day 18 (early villous stage) and appears more intense on Day 26 (villous stage), suggesting that prostasin may play roles in glandular secretion, endometrial matrix remodeling, early development of the villus, and trophoblast cell invasion. The cognate serpin-class inhibitor of prostasin, protease nexin-1 (PN-1), inhibits prostasin protease activity irreversibly but is not co-expressed with prostasin in the tissues examined. This may create a tissue environment favorable for the proteolytic activities of prostasin during the early pregnancy events. On the contrary, the reversible prostasin inhibitors, HAI-1 and HAI-2, may have a role in this setting. The reversible inhibition could provide a dynamitic control for the interactions among prostasin protease and its substrates and inhibitors.

In 2007, Zhang and colleagues[6] investigated the prostasin expression in rhesus monkey ovary during the menstrual cycle and early pregnancy, focusing on the ovarian follicle development and corpus luteum (CL) formation. Based on the localization of prostasin in the pre-ovulatory dominant follicles and in the corpus luteum after ovulation, it is speculated that prostasin may be involved in follicular growth and ovulation, and matrix degradation and remodeling during CL formation. In addition, prostasin may modulate corpus luteum formation and maintenance during early pregnancy. Interestingly, in contrast to the lack of prostasin and PN-1 co-expression in the implanting embryo, PN-1 is coordinately localized with prostasin in the ovary and corpus luteal cells during the menstrual cycle and early pregnancy.

In 2009, Ma and colleagues[7] investigated the prostasin expression in human placentas at different gestational stages. The immunoreactive prostasin is found at high levels in various trophoblasts including the villous cytotrophoblast, the syncytiotrophoblast, the column cytotrophoblast, as well as the invasive extravillous trophoblast in early pregnancy during gestation weeks 6–7, and the expression is decreased gradually to the full term.

In 2005, an effort to establish a constitutive prostasin germline knockout (KO) mouse yielded a negative result. A neo[r] gene was inserted to disrupt the mouse prostasin gene (*Prss8*) and the hemizygote prostasin-KO mice were produced (Chao, unpublished results, Medical University of South Carolina, USA). However, when the hemizygotes were crossed to obtain the homozygote prostasin-KO mice, among a total of 130 mice genotyped at weaning, none were confirmed to be a homozygote prostasin-KO (Chai, unpublished results, University of Central Florida, USA). The failure to produce a germline homozygote prostasin-KO mouse indicated that the gene inactivation is embryonic lethal.

In 2013, Hummler and colleagues[8] reported that a constitutive germline knockout of the prostasin gene in the mouse leads to a defective placenta development and the embryos die before E14.5 (embryonic day 14.5). To generate the constitutive germline prostasin–KO mice, hemizygous CAP1/*Prss8*[Δ/+] animals were crossed. No homozygote prostasin-KO mice could be identified at weaning. Examination of the embryos from E8.5–16.5 revealed that no homozygote prostasin-KO embryos survived past E14.5 while the embryos surviving on E12.5 had no obvious developmental defects in neural tube closure nor heart malformations. However, a reduced vascular development and an incomplete placental cellular maturation were observed in the tissues lacking the prostasin gene. The placenta appeared pale and lacked the arborescence of vessels referred to as the cotyledons. The cotyledons are the functional units of the placenta separated by the placental septa. Each cotyledon has a main chorionic villus with many branches and subbranches. The cotyledons are surrounded by the maternal blood and receive the fetal blood via chorionic villus capillaries from the chorionic vessels. It is with these connections, oxygen and nutrients are exchanged between the embryos/fetus and the mother.

The most profound finding in this study was that the syncytiotrophoblast is absent at the implantation site in the homozygote prostasin-KO placenta. The expression of the mouse prostasin was surveyed in the normal animals and was found in the placenta during the period of E11.5–16.5, overlapping with the period when the trophoblast lineage is defined (E10.5–12.5) (Figure 11-2). The trophoblast gives rise to the cytotrophoblast and the syncytiotrophoblast. The cytotrophoblast cells proliferate, and some of them will differentiate, lose the nuclei, and fuse together to become the syncytiotrophoblast. The absence of the syncytiotrophoblast in the prostasin-KO placentas suggests that prostasin is required in the trophoblast transition to syncytium, i.e., having a functional role in trophoblast cell proliferation, differentiation, and fusion.

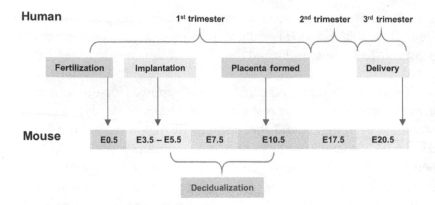

Figure 11-2. The embryonic developmental course of humans versus mice[9,10].

Further support to this hypothesis came in 2016, when Fu and colleagues[11] investigated on prostasin's function using an established human trophoblast cell line (B6Tert-1) and found that prostasin regulates the proliferation of the B6Tert-1 cells via the EGF-EGFR signaling pathway.

The syncytiotrophoblast is responsible for making the connection of the fetal blood network with the maternal blood. When the syncytiotrophoblast is not well formed, the remodeling of the maternal blood vessel is impeded, resulting in inadequate blood vessel formation during placental maturation. If the placenta does not mature and function properly, the pregnancy cannot be sustained.

To provide direct evidence that the embryonic lethality associated with the prostasin-KO is due to the placental maturation failure, Hummler and colleagues[8] created another transgenic line in which the prostasin gene is inactivated in the epiblast but not in the trophoblast. The epiblast is the foundation of the embryo whereas the trophoblast is the foundation of the placenta. The *Sox2::Cre*[Tg/+] transgenic mice were used for generating the epiblast-specific conditional mutation. In these mice, the Cre recombinase is under the control of the *Sox2* (SRY-box containing gene 2) promoter, which directs its specific expression in the epiblast of pre-implantation embryos. Male CAP1/*Prss8*[Δ/+];*Sox2::Cre*[Tg/+] mice were crossed with CAP1/*Prss8*[lox/lox] females to generate the embryo-specific prostasin-KO animals. At E14.5, the embryos without the prostasin gene were alive and had no morphological differences when compared to the controls. The placentas of these mice expressed prostasin and developed to maturity, supporting the embryo development to term. However, these mice die shortly after birth due to a skin defect (hyperkeratosis) and dehydration associated with the absence of prostasin in the skin, probably due to the *Sox2* promoter activity in the neonatal skin[12]. The skin phenotype in these mice is similar to that described by the same research group earlier in 2005[13]. In the earlier study, the prostasin gene was specifically silenced in the skin and mice died within 60 hours after birth.

Pregnancy is a physiological process but can become a pathophysiological process if it is not regulated correctly, resulting in hypertensive complications such as preeclampsia, pregnancy-induced hypertension (PIH), or maternal chronic hypertension.

In 2015, Yang and colleagues[14] examined prostasin expression by means of immunohistochemistry and reported that the expression is increased in the placental syncytiotrophoblasts of patients with early-onset severe preeclampsia. The proposed mechanism is that prostasin suppressed the invasion process in preeclampsia by attenuating the secretion of matrix metalloproteases MMP2 and MMP9. A shallow trophoblast invasion leads to an impaired remodeling of the uterine spiral arteries, potentially leading to placental ischemia. In another study by Frederiksen-Møller and colleagues[15], prostasin expression was found unchanged by means of western blotting and ELISA in samples of total placenta homogenates from patients with preeclampsia when compared to the control samples. The urinary, but not the blood prostasin content, was found to be higher in the patients versus the controls.

Once again, as we have seen in the functional study of prostasin in tight junction formation and maintenance, it appears that the appropriate prostasin protein quantity may also be essential in the trophoblast cells as too much or not enough of it would lead to inadequate placentation. Whether prostasin plays a role in regulating the tight junction in the trophoblast cells *in vivo* as it does in the skin, in addition to regulating trophoblast proliferation and differentiation, is not clear at the present time. However, this hypothesis is supported by an *in vitro* study. In 2015, Chai and colleagues[16] reported that in the B6Tert-1 human trophoblast cells, the level of the prostasin protein was positively correlated with the cell-cell tight junction formation and in the same cells, it can also be negatively correlated. When the prostasin expression was induced to a level at up to 4.5-fold higher over the baseline in the tet-regulated expression system established in these cells, the tight junctions were increasing as measured by the transepithelial electrical resistance, which increased with the amount of prostasin. When the prostasin expression was induced to beyond this level and up to a 9-fold overall increase, the tight junctions could not be formed or maintained. The absence of prostasin is embryonic lethal during reproduction, but an over-abundance of prostasin is also detrimental to the epithelial integrity.

Cumulative research data have implicated prostasin for a plethora of functional roles in both placenta formation and tumor formation. Prostasin is most likely an inhibitor in epithelial cell proliferation, migration, and invasion, but a promotor in epithelial cell differentiation. In contrast, prostasin may promote trophoblast cell proliferation via the EGF-EGFR pathway[9]. One important lesson that stands out from many experimental models to assess the function of prostasin is that the proper expression level of prostasin is key to its function in the different tissue and cellular contexts. What is the "just right" amount of prostasin may be a challenging topic in the consideration of developing prostasin as a therapeutic agent.

In reality, the placenta is a temporary non-self organ to a woman during pregnancy. The formation of the placenta is very much like the formation of tumors, both involve inflammation, invasion, angiogenesis, and immune tolerance or escape. However, the normal growth of a placenta is precisely pre-programed and a well-controlled process once the zygote is formed, and the placenta is repelled from the uterus at the delivery of the fetus. Tumors, on the other hand, can happen anywhere in the body without pre-programing for the initiation and the progression.

It is evident that the investigation of prostasin's involvement in human reproduction produced a great deal of information on the female side of the business but the question that we asked at the start of this chapter remained open and unaddressed. What is the significance

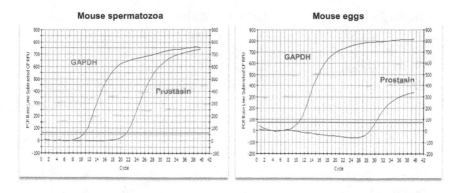

Figure 11-3. Revere-transcription and quantitative polymerase chain reaction (RT-qPCR) analysis of mouse prostasin mRNA expression. The prostasin mRNA level in mouse eggs is only about 0.3% of that in the sperm.

of prostasin in the semen? First, isolated mouse sperm have prostasin mRNA, which could be part of the leftover mRNAs from before the meiotic division. Second, the ejaculated sperm are soaked in the prostasin-rich seminal plasma where the prostasome-bound prostasin may be able to fuse or coat on the sperm membrane, perhaps helping the sperm escape immune surveillance. Conversely, mouse eggs produced from super-ovulation have very little prostasin mRNA, if any (Figure 11-3). It is speculated that during the first few days, a zygote and the early-stage blastocytes may depend on that preexisting prostasin for proper functions until the embryo makes enough of its own prostasin following the embryonic epigenetic reprogramming.

References

1. Hunkapiller NM, Gasperowicz M, Kapidzic M, Plaks V, Maltepe E, Kitajewski J, Cross JC, Fisher SJ (2011). A role for Notch signaling in trophoblast endovascular invasion and in the pathogenesis of pre-eclampsia. *Development*. 138(14):2987–2998.
2. Graham CH, Lala PK (1992). Mechanisms of placental invasion of the uterus and their control. *Biochem Cell Biol*. 70(10-11):867–874.
3. Karmakar S, Das C (2002). Regulation of trophoblast invasion by IL-1beta and TGF-beta1. *Am J Reprod Immunol*. 48(4):210–219.

4. Tuyen DG, Kitamura K, Adachi M, Miyoshi T, Wakida N, Nagano J, Nonoguchi H, Tomita K (2005). Inhibition of prostasin expression by TGF-beta1 in renal epithelial cells. *Kidney Int.* 67(1):193–200.

5. Lin HY, Zhang H, Yang Q, Wang HX, Wang HM, Chai KX, Chen LM, Zhu C (2006). Expression of prostasin and protease nexin-1 in rhesus monkey (Macaca mulatta) endometrium and placenta during early pregnancy. *J Histochem Cytochem.* 54(10):1139–1147.

6. Zhang H, Lin HY, Yang Q, Wang HX, Chai KX, Chen LM, Zhu C (2007). Expression of prostasin serine protease and protease nexin-1 (PN-1) in rhesus monkey ovary during menstrual cycle and early pregnancy. *J Histochem Cytochem.* 55(12):1237–1244.

7. Ma XJ, Fu YY, Li YX, Chen LM, Chai K, Wang YL (2009). Prostasin inhibits cell invasion in human choriocarcinomal JEG-3 cells. *Histochem Cell Biol.* 132(6):639–646.

8. Hummler E, Dousse A, Rieder A, Stehle JC, Rubera I, Osterheld MC, Beermann F, Frateschi S, Charles RP (2013). The channel-activating protease CAP1/Prss8 is required for placental labyrinth maturation. *PLoS One.* 8(2):e55796.

9. Sones JL, Davisson RL (2016). Preeclampsia, of mice and women. *Physiol Genomics.* 48(8):565–572.

10. Blum JL, Chen LC, Zelikoff JT (2017). Exposure to ambient particulate matter during specific gestational periods produces adverse obstetric consequences in mice. *Environ Health Perspect.* 125(7):077020.

11. Fu YY, Gao WL, Chen M, Chai KX, Wang YL, Chen LM (2010). Prostasin regulates human placental trophoblast cell proliferation via the epidermal growth factor receptor signaling pathway. *Hum Reprod.* 25(3):623–632.

12. Lesko MH, Driskell RR, Kretzschmar K, Goldie SJ, Watt FM (2013). Sox2 modulates the function of two distinct cell lineages in mouse skin. *Dev Biol.* 382(1):15–26.

13. Leyvraz C, Charles RP, Rubera I, Guitard M, Rotman S, Breiden B, Sandhoff K, Hummler E (2005). The epidermal barrier function is dependent on the serine protease CAP1/Prss8. *J Cell Biol.* 170(3): 487–496.

14. Yang Y, Zhang J, Gong Y, Liu X, Bai Y, Xu W, Zhou R (2015). Increased expression of prostasin contributes to early-onset severe preeclampsia through inhibiting trophoblast invasion. *J Perinatol.* 35(1):16–22.

15. Frederiksen-Møller B, Jørgensen JS, Hansen MR, Krigslund O, Vogel LK, Andersen LB, Jensen BL (2016). Prostasin and matriptase (ST14) in placenta from preeclamptic and healthy pregnant women. *J Hypertens.* 34(2):298–306.

16. Chai AC, Robinson AL, Chai KX, Chen LM (2015). Ibuprofen regulates the expression and function of membrane-associated serine proteases prostasin and matriptase. *BMC Cancer.* 15:1025.

Chapter 12

Prostasin in Inflammation and Infection

Hematopoietic immune cells are the principal cells of the host defense. The immune cells are inside the circulatory system and travel with the blood, a tissue, and a fluid enclosed inside the blood vessels. How do the immune cells know when and how to protect the body from and fight against the foreign agents of harm? One way is through the interactions with the epithelial cells. The epithelial cells cover the external and the internal surfaces of the body and are the first defense boundary against environmental insults and the first responders to the invaders. The internal surfaces such as that of the lungs and the gastrointestinal (GI) tract are topologically "external", in a continuum with the skin. The epithelial cells can be viewed as signaling hubs which integrate signals from the outside to the inside (outside-in) or the inside to the outside (inside-out) by communicating with the surrounding cells and soluble factors. A compromise of the epithelial physical protection elicits an innate immune response, accompanied by the gene expression and secretory changes. This is often referred to as an inflammation response. The secreted soluble factors, collectively referred to as cytokines, cooperate with the immune cells infiltrating to the site of compromise and a complex molecular and cellular program of neutralizing the foreign agents and repairing the compromised epithelium would ensue.

Epithelial inflammation is a defense mechanism in response to the harmful insults and is an event critical to maintaining the epithelial homeostasis. In the process of tissue injury and remodeling, the epithelial cells die, and the activated epithelial stem cells proliferate and differentiate. Many serine proteases are up-regulated or activated during epithelial inflammation, e.g., the human airway trypsin-like protease (HAT), a human airway type-II transmembrane serine protease (TTSP) which cleaves and activates the hemagglutinin antigen (HA) of the influenza virus, promoting viral infection[1]. This is an ironic example of a host cell membrane serine protease being hijacked by an infectious agent to enhance its own entry into the host cells. In the past few years, such a mechanism has been highlighted unfortunately by the entry of the severe acute respiratory syndrome coronavirus 2 (SARS-CoV-2) into the epithelial cells, utilizing the host membrane proteases angiotensin-converting enzyme 2 (ACE2) and transmembrane serine protease 2 (TMPRSS2).

On the contrary, prostasin is reported to decrease Dengue virus replication and propagation via down-regulating the epidermal growth factor receptor (EGFR) expression[2]. Prostasin has an almost universal presence in the epithelia and is presented on the apical side of the epithelial cells, well positioned to interact with any foreign agents. A role for prostasin in the innate immunity of the epithelium was investigated first in the bladder.

The human urine ranks second as a biological source rich in the prostasin protein, at a concentration about 2 µg/ml[3]. The origin of prostasin in the urine could be traced back to epithelial cells anywhere in the urinary tract including the kidney and the bladder. A urinary tract infection (UTI) is an infection of the urinary system including the kidney, ureter, bladder, and urethra. It is an exceedingly common worldwide problem, affecting women more so than men at a ratio of 30:1 with 1 in 5 adult women to experience UTI at some point of life. Most UTI cases are caused by *Escherichia coli*, a Gram-negative bacterium normally living in the intestines of healthy people. The pathogenic component of Gram-negative bacteria, the lipopolysaccharide (LPS) activates the innate immune program via the toll-like receptor 4 (TLR4), a member of the pattern recognition receptor family[4,5]. TLR4 also recognizes other pathogen-associated molecular patterns (PAMPs). TLR4 in complex with MD-2 (myeloid differentiation factor 2, or lymphocyte antigen 96 encoded by the *LY96* gene) and CD14 (cluster of differentiation 14) mediates the signal transduction upon LPS stimulation.

TLR4 is expressed as a transmembrane protein mostly in the myeloid cells such as the erythrocytes, granulocytes, and macrophages, but is also expressed in some epithelial cells, e.g., the bladder epithelial cells[6], called the urothelial cells.

In 2006, Chen and colleagues[7] investigated the molecular and functional changes with a keen focus on prostasin in the mouse bladder under inflammation induced by LPS. Two mouse models were used in the study, one was a transgenic model over-expressing the human prostasin ubiquitously, while the second involved lipid-assisted gene delivery to express the human prostasin in the mouse bladder *in situ*. The transgenic mouse expressing the human prostasin had a full-length human prostasin cDNA under the control of the Rous Sarcoma virus (RSV) long-terminal repeat. This model was generated by the conventional method using microinjection of the linearized prostasin cDNA plasmid into the FVB-strain mouse embryos, performed by the ESCore Facility of the University of Cincinnati for Dr. Julie Chao at the Medical University of South Carolina (MUSC, USA). The transgenic mice were screened, verified for the genomic integration of the transgene and its expression, and bred for subsequent experiments. To transiently express the human prostasin in the mouse bladder, a complex of the prostasin-expressing plasmid and liposome was delivered into the bladder via a transurethral catheter. Mice from both models were challenged with intraperitoneal injection of LPS to induce bladder inflammation over a period of 18 hours.

Expression of the mouse prostasin was confirmed in the urothelium by means of immunohistochemistry (IHC) and reverse transcription/quantitative polymerase chain reaction (RT-qPCR). Expression of the transgenic human prostasin in the mouse bladder was confirmed by western blot and RT-qPCR. The bladder inflammation was confirmed by the induced expression of the signature proteins and cytokines responding to an LPS stimulation. Among them, the inducible nitric oxide synthase (iNOS), cyclooxygenase-2 (COX2), interferon gamma (IFNγ), tumor necrosis factor alpha (TNFα), interleukin-1beta (IL-1β) and interleukin-6 (IL-6) were all robustly up-regulated in the bladder of the LPS-treated non-transgenic mice, as compared to the control mice without the LPS treatment.

The endogenous mouse prostasin mRNA was down-regulated in the bladder by the LPS treatment. This was true for the non-transgenic control FVB mice and the two independent transgenic lines with different levels of the human prostasin transgene mRNA and protein expression in the mouse urothelium. It is unexpected to see that the urothelial prostasin expression is negatively impacted during an acute inflammation, while prostasin has always been viewed as a player in epithelial cell differentiation as described in the previous chapters. The simplest and most direct interpretation, although not clear with the mechanisms, would be that the naturally evolved and adapted acute innate immune response needs prostasin to be absent.

Then the question is to see what impact a forced prostasin expression would impose on the urothelial inflammation. In the experiments described above, the human prostasin transgene expressed in the mouse urothelium in either the transgenic animals or the DNA-lipid infused animals was driven by a viral promoter not affected by the epithelial inflammation. In the transgenic mice expressing a high level of the human prostasin, the iNOS up-regulation by LPS was attenuated, with a level at only ~40% of that in the LPS-treated non-transgenic control mice. This attenuation was also observed in the mouse bladder transiently expressing the human prostasin via DNA-lipid gene delivery. The gene delivery model permitted an easy and economical way to ask the question whether the prostasin serine protease activity is required for a role in regulating epithelial inflammation. Using this method, it was shown that the iNOS up-regulation by LPS was blunted by a forced expression of the wild-type prostasin but not by a protease-inactive prostasin variant, in which the active site serine was replaced by an alanine. Further evidence of a role in regulating iNOS expression by prostasin was provided by the same research group in 2009[8]. By knocking down prostasin gene expression using small interfering RNA (siRNA), the iNOS expression was up-regulated in the BPH-1 human benign prostatic hyperplasia cell line, possibly via the regulation of the protease-activated receptor-2 (PAR-2) signaling pathway. The iNOS is an essential enzyme in the epithelial innate immune response, producing a locally concentrated supply of nitric oxide (NO), as an anti-microbial and a tumoricidal agent. Prostasin has a negative regulation effect on iNOS expression thus it must be down-regulated during the early phase of the epithelial inflammation to allow the proper iNOS induction.

The mechanisms of the LPS-induced up-regulation of iNOS expression have been studied in many cell types. The initial induction is believed to be mediated through the activation of the TLR4 complex. Subsequently, the downstream master regulator NF-κB signaling pathway is activated resulting in the first phase of the proinflammatory cytokine gene expression. Then, the immune cells are recruited and infiltrate in the inflammation site in response to the induced cytokines. This positive feedback regulation allows the second-phase cytokine gene expression by the infiltrating immune cells to produce a large amount of cytokines. Perhaps reducing the cellular prostasin abundance during the early phase of inflammation can also assist the immune cell infiltration by increasing the intercellular permeability through dissolving the cell-cell tight junction, as prostasin is known to be functionally involved in these events. In the second phase, the transcription factor interferon regulatory factor 1 (IRF-1) stimulated by IFNγ is required to enhance the high-level iNOS up-regulation[9,10]. Interestingly, the up-regulation of IFNγ expression by LPS in the prostasin transgenic mouse bladder is blunted as well. It is not clear at what stage or phase of the inflammatory response prostasin attenuated the iNOS up-regulation but very possibly, prostasin played a role in the communication between the epithelial cells and the immune cells.

Another example for a potential function of prostasin in regulating the communication of the immune cells and the epithelial cells was recorded in the study by Chen and colleagues[11] in 2021, in which they showed that over-expressing prostasin in the Calu-3 human non-small-cell lung adenocarcinoma cells up-regulates the IFNγ-induced programmed death-ligand 1 (PD-L1) expression. The up-regulated PD-L1 protein in the cancer cells could be used as a mechanism to evade immune surveillance.

The NO production in a bacterial-infected bladder is usually produced by the iNOS in the late-phase when most of the invading bacteria are cleared[12]. The NO would then have roles in urothelial cell apoptosis and shedding, which are beneficial in defending against bacterial infection and removing dead cells. However, it may function unfavorably in the late phase by interfering with urothelial cell differentiation in the renewal process[13]. Prostasin has been implicated for functional roles in epithelial differentiation, but the mouse urothelial prostasin gene expression is greatly down-regulated during the LPS-induced inflammation. The *in situ* down-regulation of prostasin in the inflamed urothelial cells would intensify and prolong the iNOS expression for the positive and beneficial effects of NO to be present in the bladder urothelium microenvironment. Nonetheless, this state must not be allowed to perpetuate or last for too long as a lack of the proper amount of prostasin would impede urothelial repair and differentiation. Thus, the urothelial prostasin expression is expected to return during the closing stages of tissue repair and differentiation. At present there is no report on the time course of prostasin expression restoration in the urothelium following an inflammatory response, but a proper look in the future is highly warranted. Prostasin may be a protective agent during the bladder inflammation by regulating the long-term NO production via reducing the iNOS expression in the urothelial cells, promoting the healing process. The reduction of prostasin expression during inflammation could potentiate iNOS up-regulation, but the action can be partially rescued in cells over-expressing prostasin, as in the case of the prostasin transgenic mice and the prostasin gene therapy model. These experimental results may have a physiological or clinical relevance in the context of chronic inflammation or cancers that result from a chronically inflamed state.

The precise molecular mechanism by which prostasin expression is greatly reduced during inflammation is not clear. It is possible that the NF-κB/Rel and IκBa signaling pathways and/or the transcription suppressor Slug are involved in suppressing the prostasin promoter activity[14,15]. The NF-κB axis is activated in bladder inflammation by the inflammatory cytokines such as TNFα[16], and the activated NF-κB can up-regulate Slug expression. The latter is a repressor of prostasin expression. The induction of TNFα expression by LPS in the mouse bladder was unaffected by the forced human prostasin transgene expression, therefore, the endogenous mouse prostasin expression down-regulation by LPS was not protected by the human prostasin transgene.

Inflammation-induced prostasin expression down-regulation was further evaluated in the mouse gastrointestinal tract by Buzza and colleagues[17] in 2017. It was reported that both the prostasin mRNA and protein expression levels were reduced in the distal colon as early as 1.5 days, preceding the clinical symptoms, after a treatment with dextran sulfate sodium (DSS), which is a well-known chemical reagent for inducing experimental colitis in mice.

Prostasin gene expression can be up-regulated by non-steroidal anti-inflammatory drugs (NSAIDs) in bladder urothelial cells as reported by Chai and colleagues[18] in 2015. The NSAIDs would have a multitude of molecular mediators but at least for the expression of prostasin the effect can be considered as beneficial. The increased presence of prostasin would be able to participate in the formation and maintenance of the epithelial tight junction, as was shown in the B6Tert-1 human trophoblast cells. The expression of prostasin in these immortalized human trophoblast cells increased the transepithelial electrical resistance (TEER) when the cells were grown to confluence, indicating the proper formation of the tight junctions. These cells are specialized epithelial cells in the placenta and possess the molecular programs necessary for the examination of a role for prostasin in the formation of the tight junction. With the current absence of a proper urothelial cell line that can provide the tool for demonstrating this phenotype, the observation from the B6Tert-1 cells can lend support to such a role for prostasin in the urothelium.

In 2014, Uchimura and colleagues[19] reported that a deletion of the prostasin gene in the mouse liver rendered the mouse sensitive to an LPS challenge. Silencing prostasin expression by siRNA in the HepG2 human hepatocarcinoma cells increases TLR4 expression, while an over-expression of prostasin reduces the TLR4 level as a result of its proteolytic cleavage, with the release of the TLR4 ectodomain into the culture medium. Consequently, the inflammatory signaling cascade through TLR4 is reduced in the cells over-expressing prostasin.

Another example of prostasin down-regulation in an inflammation state involving the expression of TLR4 was reported in 2020. Sugitani and colleagues[20] investigated prostasin expression in the inflamed mucosa of patients with inflammatory bowel disease (IBD) and suggested that prostasin has an anti-inflammation function via a down-regulation of the TLR4 signaling pathway. Immunoreactive prostasin is localized at the apical surface of the colonic mucosa of healthy individuals, but the expression is greatly reduced in the active mucosa in patients with either ulcerative colitis or Crohn's disease.

In a mouse model ($Prss8^{\Delta IEC}$) in which the prostasin gene is deleted in the cells of the intestinal tract, the colonic epithelial cells appeared to have the normal histology at least for the first 6–8 weeks after birth. This phenotype would suggest that the reduced prostasin expression seen in the inflamed colon mucosa may be secondary to and a response of the inflammation but not the initiator of the IBD. However, the absence of prostasin can exacerbate the disease conditions manifested in this animal model with an induced colitis. Colitis induced with dextran sodium sulfate presented worse phenotypes in the $Prss8^{\Delta IEC}$ mice lacking prostasin expression as compared to the $Prss8^{lox/lox}$ control mice with the proper prostasin expression. The phenotypes observed included lower body weight, severely disrupted epithelial cells, and more infiltration of the inflammatory cells in the intestinal epithelial cells in the mice without prostasin.

At the molecular level, the TLR4 expression is strongly up-regulated in the $Prss8^{\Delta IEC}$ mice and is further up-regulated by the DSS treatment. Consequently, NF-αB activation, the downstream signaling pathway of TLR4 activation, and the inflammatory cytokine expression appear pronounced in the colonic epithelial cells of the $Prss8^{\Delta IEC}$ mice.

Interestingly, the exacerbation effect can be completely suppressed by antibiotic treatment. If mice are given a broad-spectrum antibiotic for four weeks prior to the DSS induction of colitis, no difference of disease severity is observed between those expressing and those not expressing prostasin in the colon. The epithelial cell lining damage in the colon by the chemical DSS permits the entry of the luminal organisms or their associated products into the lamina propria where the innate and adaptive immunoreactions are triggered, leading to the dissemination of pro-inflammatory intestinal contents into the underlying tissue. In this case, the antibiotic could have suppressed the commensal microflora to stop the LPS-stimulated TLR4 activation.

   The current evidence supports the view that a compromised colonic epithelial mucosa barrier, either genetically, chemically, physically, or immunologically, is the primary cause of inflammatory bowel disease. The initial colitis increases TLR4 expression and activation, which then further exacerbates the disease course in the presence of the commensal microflora or in the absence of prostasin expression. It is worth noting that the tight junction protein expression and mucosal permeability to FITC-dextran are affected in the DSS-induced colitis but not worsened in the *Prss8*$^{\Delta IEC}$ mice with no colonic prostasin expression. The control mice express a minimal level of TLR4 in the colon epithelial cells, but the TLR4 expression is greatly increased when the prostasin gene is deleted, a condition further enhanced in the DSS-induced colitis. Similar results were also observed by Uchimura and colleagues in 2014[19] in the mouse liver, where a high-fat diet suppressed prostasin expression, leading to an increased TLR4 expression level.

   The DSS-induced colitis is reversible, and it would be extremely curious to learn about the molecular time course in the reversion with regard to a restoration of prostasin expression. It would also be even more curious to learn if the DSS-induced colitis is no longer reversible in the mice with the prostasin gene ablation in the colon. These questions will hopefully prompt future research to help delineate a clearer picture of prostasin's functional involvement in the colon or other epithelia during an acute inflammation and how that picture changes in a chronic inflammatory state. A hint may be taken from the loss of prostasin in the epithelial cancers, almost exclusively due to an epigenetic mechanism while no cases of genetic mutations have been reported. The colon or any other epithelium is constantly under the threat of external insults and injuries. A loss of prostasin at the gene level would spell a disaster, as was seen in the exacerbation of colitis of the prostasin-ablated mice.

   The overarching theme at the present time on prostasin and inflammation is its role in the regulation of TLR4 expression and function. Prostasin directly cleaves the TLR4 protein, thus its own down-regulation during inflammation permits TLR4 functions in response to the LPS challenge, as suggested by the results from the research on the urothelium, and supported by that in the intestinal epithelial cells with the prostasin gene knockout. The molecular mechanism of the TLR4 expression up-regulation associated with a prostasin down-regulation is unclear. It should be emphasized that other molecules interacting with prostasin, such as growth factor receptors of the receptor tyrosine kinase (RTK) and the protease-activated receptor (PAR) families may also have a role in mediating prostasin's actions in epithelial inflammation and innate immunity. These very important molecular pathways may also hold the key to the TLR4 expression up-regulation when the prostasin expression is reduced or absent.

References

1. Böttcher E, Matrosovich T, Beyerle M, Klenk HD, Garten W, Matrosovich M (2006). Proteolytic activation of influenza viruses by serine proteases TMPRSS2 and HAT from human airway epithelium. *J Virol.* 80(19):9896–9898.
2. Lin CK, Tseng CK, Wu YH, Lin CY, Huang CH, Wang WH, Liaw CC, Chen YH, Lee JC (2019). Prostasin impairs epithelial growth factor receptor activation to suppress dengue virus propagation. *J Infect Dis.* 219(9):1377–1388.
3. Yu JX, Chao L, Chao J (1994). Prostasin is a novel human serine proteinase from seminal fluid. Purification, tissue distribution, and localization in prostate gland. *J Biol Chem.* 269(29):18843–18848.
4. Vaure C, Liu Y (2014). A comparative review of toll-like receptor 4 expression and functionality in different animal species. *Front Immunol.* 5:316.
5. Brubaker SW, Bonham KS, Zanoni I, Kagan JC (2015). Innate immune pattern recognition: A cell biological perspective. *Annu Rev Immunol.* 33:257–290.
6. Bäckhed F, Meijer L, Normark S, Richter-Dahlfors A (2002). TLR4-dependent recognition of lipopolysaccharide by epithelial cells requires sCD14. *Cell Microbiol.* 4(8):493–501.
7. Chen LM, Wang C, Chen M, Marcello MR, Chao J, Chao L, Chai KX (2006). Prostasin attenuates inducible nitric oxide synthase expression in lipopolysaccharide-induced urinary bladder inflammation. *Am J Physiol Renal Physiol.* 291(3):F567–F577.
8. Chen LM, Hatfield ML, Fu YY, Chai KX (2009). Prostasin regulates iNOS and cyclin D1 expression by modulating protease-activated receptor-2 signaling in prostate epithelial cells. *Prostate.* 69(16):1790–1801.

9. Kamijo R, Harada H, Matsuyama T, Bosland M, Gerecitano J, Shapiro D, Le J, Koh SI, Kimura T, Green SJ (1994). Requirement for transcription factor IRF-1 in NO synthase induction in macrophages. *Science.* 263(5153):1612–1615.

10. Martin E, Nathan C, Xie QW (1994). Role of interferon regulatory factor 1 in induction of nitric oxide synthase. *J Exp Med.* 180(3):977–984.

11. Chen LM, Chai JC, Liu B, Strutt TM, McKinstry KK, Chai KX (2021). Prostasin regulates PD-L1 expression in human lung cancer cells. *Biosci Rep.* 41(7):BSR20211370.

12. Poljakovic M, Svensson ML, Svanborg C, Johansson K, Larsson B, Persson K (2001). Escherichia coli-induced inducible nitric oxide synthase and cyclooxygenase expression in the mouse bladder and kidney. *Kidney Int.* 59(3):893–904.

13. Elgavish A, Robert B, Lloyd K, Reed R (1996). Nitric oxide mediates the action of lipoteichoic acid on the function of human urothelial cells. *J Cell Physiol.* 169(1):66–77.

14. Tuyen DG, Kitamura K, Adachi M, Miyoshi T, Wakida N, Nagano J, Nonoguchi H, Tomita K (2005). Inhibition of prostasin expression by TGF-beta1 in renal epithelial cells. *Kidney Int.* 67(1):193–200.

15. Chen M, Chen LM, Chai KX (2006). Androgen regulation of prostasin gene expression is mediated by sterol-regulatory element-binding proteins and SLUG. *Prostate.* 66(9):911–920.

16. Fu YY, Nergard JC, Barnette NK, Wang YL, Chai KX, Chen LM (2012). Proteasome inhibition augments cigarette smoke-induced GM-CSF expression in trophoblast cells via the epidermal growth factor receptor. *PLoS One.* 7(8):e43042.

17. Buzza MS, Johnson TA, Conway GD, Martin EW, Mukhopadhyay S, Shea-Donohue T, Antalis TM (2017). Inflammatory cytokines down-regulate the barrier-protective prostasin-matriptase proteolytic cascade early in experimental colitis. *J Biol Chem.* 292(26):10801–10812.

18. Chai AC, Robinson AL, Chai KX, Chen LM (2015). Ibuprofen regulates the expression and function of membrane-associated serine proteases prostasin and matriptase. *BMC Cancer.* 15:1025.

19. Uchimura K, Hayata M, Mizumoto T, Miyasato Y, Kakizoe Y, Morinaga J, Onoue T, Yamazoe R, Ueda M, Adachi M, Miyoshi T, Shiraishi N, Ogawa W, Fukuda K, Kondo T, Matsumura T, Araki E, Tomita K, Kitamura K (2014). The serine protease prostasin regulates hepatic insulin sensitivity by modulating TLR4 signalling. *Nat Commun.* 5:3428.

20. Sugitani Y, Nishida A, Inatomi O, Ohno M, Imai T, Kawahara M, Kitamura K, Andoh A (2020). Sodium absorption stimulator prostasin (PRSS8) has an anti-inflammatory effect via downregulation of TLR4 signaling in inflammatory bowel disease. *J Gastroenterol.* 55(4):408–417.

Chapter 13

Prostasin in Other Organs

Prostasin has always been described in the literature as an epithelial membrane-anchored extracellular serine protease. The first expression profiling by means of reverse transcription and polymerase chain reaction (RT-PCR) and Southern hybridization using three prostasin-specific oligonucleotides did not detect the human prostasin mRNA transcript in the atrium, ventricle, aorta, vein, artery, or the human umbilical vein endothelial cells (HUVEC), lymphocytes, polymorphonuclear cells (PMNC). Also negative for the human prostasin mRNA transcript in this experiment were the testis, ovary, uterus, spleen, brain cortex, and muscle. All epithelial tissues examined were positive including the prostate, salivary glands, kidney, lung, colon, bronchus, along with the liver, pancreas, the human kidney proximal tubule, and the LNCaP human prostate cancer cell line[1]. In an early gene atlas of the human protein-coding transcriptome analysis of 79 tissues, the trachea, thyroid, placenta, and small intestine were shown to express the prostasin mRNA at above the median level. In the GTEx RNA-seq gene expression analysis of 54 tissues from 17,382 samples (948 donors) (V8, Aug 2019), the cervix, esophagus, skin, stomach, and vagina were also found to express the prostasin mRNA. In the initial study that reported prostasin's isolation from the seminal plasma, the human prostasin protein was found in the prostate, colon, lung, kidney, pancreas, salivary gland, liver, and bronchus[2]. The functions of prostasin in the epithelial tissues are discussed in the other chapters. Here we will focus on some unique sites of prostasin expression or action.

13.1 The blood

In the extrinsic pathway of blood coagulation, tissue factor exposed at the injury site binds to the activated factor VII (FVIIa) in the circulation at a low basal level to initiate a conversion of more FVII zymogen to FVIIa and the subsequent coagulation cascade. In search of additional serine proteases responsible for the initial Fviia generation to quickly engage the coagulation cascade, in 2020, Khandekar and colleagues[3] performed a "piggyback knockdown"[4] of 179 zebrafish genes encoding serine protease domains using annotated sequence information from the NCBI/ENSEMBEL database. The term "piggy-backing" refers to a simultaneous knockdown of expression for many genes by gene-specific anti-sense oligonucleotide vivo-morpholinos that can enter the cell to silence gene expression[5]. The piggybacking strategy reduces the amount of testing and the positive results (hits) are then re-screened. In these experiments, the effect of gene silencing on blood clotting was monitored in a prolonged kinetic prothrombin time (kPT) assay. The assay measures the amount of fibrin formation induced by the plasma of zebrafish using the tissue factor (thrombo-plastin) pathway of activating thrombin to cleave human fibrinogen. The time to half maximal fibrin formation was used as the standard to determine if there is a phenotype associated with knocking-down a specific gene, manifested as a delay. After three rounds of screening, a delayed fibrin formation time was observed in zebrafish when the orthologue of the prostasin gene was silenced. This result suggested a reduced generation of Fviia, which was further supported by results from an ELISA showing a ~85–90% reduction of the activated Fvii (Fviia) level while the Fvii zymogen level was only reduced by ~10–15%. Prostasin was proposed as an activator for FVII (Fvii in zebrafish), either directly via a proteolytic cleavage or via other mechanisms.

The zebrafish is an *in vivo* model to study hemostasis[6], especially for validating candidate genes identified in humans via reverse genetics (gene mapping) because of the genomic homology and conservation of the blood coagulation cascades, sharing 70% of the human genes and containing all coagulating factor orthologues. The autosomal domi-nant familial thrombocytopenia in humans, a condition of low blood platelet count, was mapped to chromosome 10p[7], with the microtubule-associated serine/threonine-like kinase (*MASTL*) identified as the candidate disease gene[8]. Silencing the zebrafish *mastl* orthologue by morpholinos reproduced the human clinical phenotypes. As we have discussed earlier, the OMIM does not list any hereditary human disorder associated with a known prostasin variant. The zebrafish phenotype of reduced Fvii activation associated with a prostasin gene silencing is very robust, but it is not clear if this is also conserved in humans.

The mRNA sequence of the human prostasin zebrafish orthologue investigated in the study is zgc:92313, with the GenBank Accession Number BC076000, at 1,498 nucleotides (nt) in length. A pairwise nucleotide sequence alignment with the human prostasin mRNA, Accession Number NM_002773 (1,837 nt), revealed a 48.99% shared identity.

The translated amino acid sequences of the zebrafish prostasin and the human prostasin share 42.5% identity in a 261-residue overlap, which included both the light and heavy chains of the mature protein, with minimal gaps (1.9%). The regions around the catalytic triad residues, His/Asp/Ser, are highly conserved. There is a high degree of confidence to accept the presumed orthologue relationship between the zebrafish prostasin implicated in blood coagulation and the human prostasin (Figure 13-1).

The antisense morpholinos in the piggyback knockdown screening were injected into the blood stream of zebrafish. The zebrafish blood coagulation defect associated with the prostasin knockdown was tested out using the fish plasma, after the injection of the antisense vivo-morpholinos into the blood stream. Vivo-morpholinos by short-term intravenous delivery can achieve a tissue distribution and the expected gene expression knockdown in the liver, small intestine, colon, muscle, lung, and stomach, as well as in the spleen, heart, skin, and brain but with lesser efficiency. As we have indicated in the beginning of this chapter, the human blood cells and blood vessel cells are not known to express prostasin. The first report on the presence of prostasin protein in human blood came from a study on prostasin as a potential serum marker for ovarian cancer[9], in which the control subjects have an average serum prostasin level of 7.5 µg/mL (95% CI = 6.6–8.3 µg/mL).

```
                                  ↓
Zebrafish    21  GEAQECGRPPMINRIVGGSSAADGAWPWQVDIQGEKSKHVCGGTIISENWVLSAAHCFPN
Human        32  GAEAPCGVAPQA-RITGGSSAVAGQWPWQVSITYE-GVHVCGGSLVSEQWVLSAAHCFPS
                 *   **  *   ** ***** * ***** *  *   ***** ** **********

Zebrafish    81  PNDISGYLIYAGRQQLNGWNPDETSHRISRVVVPLGYTDPQLGQDIALVELATPFVYTER
Human        90  EHHKEAYEVKLGAHQLDSYSEDAKVSTLKDIIPHPSYLQEGSQGDIALLQLSRPITFSRY
                 *    *  **     *             *        *     **** *  *

Zebrafish   141  IQPVCLPYANVEFTSDMRCMITGWGDIREGVALQGVGPLQEVQVPIIDSQICQDMFLTN-
Human       150  IRPICLPAANASFPNGLHCTVTGWGHVAPSVSLLTPKPLQQLEVPLISRETCNCLYNIDA
                 * * *** **  *      * ****    ** *    *** ** *       *

Zebrafish   200  -PTENIDIRPDMMCAGFQQGGKDSCQGDSGGPLACQISDGSWVQAGIVSFGLGCAEANRP
Human       210  KPEEPHFVQEDMVCAGYVEGGKDACQGDSGGPLSCPV-EGLWYLTGIVSWGDACGARNRP
                   * *      ** ***    **** ********* *    * *  **** *  *  ***

Zebrafish   259  GVYAKVSSFTNFIQTHVGGIQ
Human       269  GVYTLASSYASWIQSKVTELQ
                 ***   **    **  *   *
```

Figure 13-1. Amino acid sequence alignment of the zebrafish prostasin orthologue to the human prostasin. The cleavage site for prostasin activation is indicated by the red arrow. The catalytic triad residues are shown in red font, and the sequence conservation around the triad residues is shaded green.

This was a mixed control group of 137 subjects, including 24 with other gynecologic cancers, 42 with benign gynecologic diseases, and 71 with no known gynecologic diseases. This serum concentration of prostasin is approximately 200 nM which is unusually high, while the FVII zymogen is at approximately 500 ng/mL or 10 nM[10].

Recently, it has been reported that the extracellular vesicles known as the exosomes in human blood stream, contain prostasin, which was the most up-regulated in large extracellular vesicles (LEVs, 20,000 × g pellets) in the plasma of patients with severe COVID-19 infection when compared to healthy individuals[11]. Also significantly up-regulated in the LEVs in the severe COVID-19 plasma was tissue factor (TF, CD142). The TF up-regulation in EVs from severe COVID-19 cases was reported by another independent study that also showed the EV-surface TF being biologically active. The EVs released by cells may initiate clotting with the increased amounts of pro-coagulant factors to contribute to COVID-19 disease severity[12]. EVs released from the tumors in cancer patients have been known to contribute to thrombosis via the membrane surface TF and pro-coagulating lipids[13]. The presentation of prostasin in the exosomes was first reported in the urinary exosomes in a study of potential markers for aldosteronism[14,15]. In the EVs released from the Calu-3 human lung adenocarcinoma cells, the membrane surface prostasin was shown to be an active serine protease[16].

All these studies provide a plausible molecular mechanistic explanation of the blood coagulation defect associated with knocking down the prostasin orthologue expression via intravenous injection of antisense vivo-morpholinos in zebrafish. The organs and tissues that normally express prostasin will have a reduced expression upon the delivery of the vivo-morpholinos. This will result in a reduced amount of prostasin associated with the EVs in the circulation. On the membrane surface of the circulating EVs, the presumed active serine protease prostasin has a facilitating role to the initiation of coagulation by the TF-Fviia complex, in the step of Fvii activation to Fviia. What remains unclear is how prostasin interacts with TF or Fvii/Fviia and if the interaction requires the serine protease activity. The role of prostasin in coagulation is novel and continued research to define the interactions of this extracellular membrane serine protease with the immediately relevant molecules could potentially bring forth new ways of treating cardio-vascular diseases, e.g., stroke.

Hummler and colleagues[17] reported that knocking out (KO) the prostasin gene expression in the mouse is detrimental to placenta development. Homozygote prostasin-KO embryos cannot survive beyond embryonic day 14.5 (E14.5). Histologically, the placentae at E12.5 appeared pale, poorly vascularized, and lacked the arborescence of vessels (cotyledons). TF is present at high levels in the placenta and is required in the maintenance of the placental labyrinth and hemostasis[18,19]. It would be interesting to learn if prostasin plays a role in the vasculature formation during placentation via regulating TF and/or FVII functions.

13.2 The liver

The liver is an essential organ of the human body with many functions such as protein synthesis, metabolism of carbohydrates, proteins, amino acids, and lipids, and detoxification. The liver consists of mostly hepatocytes which are not a rich source of prostasin expression, with ~2.59 nanograms of prostasin per milligram of the total cellular protein as determined by an ELISA in the original study that identified prostasin[2]. The prostasin mRNA transcript was detected in the human liver by RT-PCR and Southern blot analysis[1], but a recent survey of gene expression by RNA-seq in 54 tissues with 17,382 samples from 948 donors (GTEx V8, Aug 2019)[20], did not show a significant amount of liver expression of the prostasin mRNA. RNA-seq is a modern method in transcriptome studies involving the next-generation (next-gen) sequencing technologies to determine the quantities and sequence variations of RNA in a tissue or cell. For the human prostasin mRNA transcript, the minor salivary gland has the highest median expression at 236.7 TPM (Transcripts Per Kilobase Million) from a sample size of 162. In the liver, the prostasin mRNA level is at only 12.14 TPM (sample size 226). We can compare these to the levels of the prostasin mRNA in the lung and the prostate, at 83.23 TPM (sample size 578) and 56.57 TPM (sample size 245) to gain some perspectives on the presence of prostasin mRNA in the liver.

In the mouse, the tissue-specific expression pattern of prostasin was analysed by List and colleagues in 2007[21]. They established an atlas of co-localization of prostasin and matriptase in mouse tissues. For viewing the matriptase expression, a knock-in mouse model (C57Bl/6J-NIH Black Swiss) was generated, in which a promoter-less β-galactosidase marker gene was inserted into one of the matriptase alleles disrupting the matriptase serine protease domain (matriptase^{+}/$^{E16\beta\text{-}gal}$ mice). By this design, the endogenous matriptase expression pattern can be viewed by X-gal staining generated by the β-galactosidase in the matriptase-β-galactosidase fusion protein. For viewing the prostasin expression pattern, a monoclonal antibody (Becton, Dickinson, and Company) was used in immunohistochemical staining of mouse tissues. In the mouse the co-expression of matriptase and prostasin is mainly in all epithelial tissues. Prostasin expression is negative in the liver and the bile duct epithelium. In our hands using a polyclonal prostasin antibody[22], prostasin expression is detected in the bile duct epithelial cells, but sparsely in mouse hepatocytes (Chen, unpublished data, University of Central Florida).

Nevertheless, mouse models with either a liver-specific prostasin over-expression or a liver-specific prostasin gene deletion were created to probe for a potential functional phenotype associated with prostasin gene or expression modifications in this organ.

In 2014, Uchimura and colleagues[23] generated a mouse model in which the mouse prostasin gene was interrupted in the liver for the purpose of investigating type 2 diabetes as a result of insulin resistance induced by long-term high-fat diet consumption. The rationale to target the prostasin gene (*Prss8* in mice) was based on prostasin's role in regulating the inflammation response induced by the bacterial lipopolysaccharides (LPS), which could activate the pattern recognition receptor toll-like receptor 4 (TLR4). TLR4 has a role in high-fat-induced insulin resistance via inflammation. The transgenic *Prss8^{lox/lox}* mice, wherein two *loxP* sites flank the prostasin gene exons 3–5 (out of the 6 exons), were crossed with the *Alb-Cre* transgenic mice with an albumin promoter-driven liver-specific Cre recombinase expression (The Jackson laboratory, Bar Harbor, ME, USA) to generate the *Alb-CrePrss8^{lox/+}* mice, which were then self-crossed to generate the liver-specific prostasin knockout mice (LKO).

The normal mouse liver did not express detectable amounts of the prostasin protein under fasting but expressed prostasin after refeeding with sucrose in mice fed with a normal diet only, not much in those fed with a high-fat diet. The attenuation of prostasin expression in the latter group was hypothesized to be caused by the endoplasmic reticulum (ER) stress induced by the high-fat diet. As expected, the high-fat diet also induced insulin resistance. It was suggested that prostasin might be involved in regulating insulin resistance, because in mice with an engineered transient prostasin over-expression in the liver, the insulin resistance was alleviated.

To further confirm prostasin's role in insulin resistance, the liver-specific prostasin KO (LKO) mice were subjected to the same experiments. The LKO mice had higher levels of fasting blood glucose and serum insulin when fed with a high-fat diet and also after sucrose refeeding. In addition, prostasin KO had an enhancement effect on the response to LPS marked by a higher expression of the LPS-stimulated cytokines. The most important finding of this study is that prostasin negatively regulates the TLR4 expression in mouse liver and the HepG2 human hepatocellular carcinoma cell line, and mediates proteolytic shedding of the TLR4 extracellular domain (ECD) when co-expressed in the HEK-293 human embryonic kidney cells.

The *db/db* mice have a spontaneous mutation (*Lepr*[db]) that causes diabetes and are often used to model type 2 diabetes and obesity. In the *db/db* mice, prostasin expression was also found to be inversely related to the TLR4 expression under the refeeding condition. In summary, type 2 diabetes induced by the high-fat diet and the postprandial endotoxemia may be related to the loss of prostasin function in the liver on regulating TLR4 expression and function.

Whereas, in 2021, Sekine and colleagues[24] generated a mouse model in which the human prostasin gene was over-expressed in the liver with the use of the mouse albumin gene promoter. These mice have lower levels of fasting blood glucose after a 14-week high-fat diet regimen, when compared with the control mice. In addition, the expression levels of genes relating to the cholesterol biosynthetic pathways were shown to be reduced following the analysis with the GeneChip Mouse Gene 2.0 ST Array (Affymetrix, Inc., Santa Clara, CA, USA). The human prostasin gene expression is up-regulated by the sterol-response element-binding proteins (SREBPs)[25], which are key regulators of genes involved in cholesterol synthesis. The reciprocal regulation of prostasin and genes of the cholesterol biosynthetic pathways merits investing in future research.

The interpretation of the transgenic mouse studies on the loss or gain of functions of liver-specific prostasin expression should be a cautious one when it concerns the relevance to human health and disease, as prostasin is by no means highly expressed in the human liver. By an approach to integrate mouse liver co-expression networks with human lipid GWAS data to identify regulators of cholesterol and lipid metabolism[26,27], prostasin emerged as one of 48 autosomal genes showing replication in mouse liver networks and association with human plasma lipid traits using the Global Lipid Genetics Consortium (GLGC) human GWAS data for plasma total cholesterol (TC), LDL-cholesterol, HDL-cholesterol, and triglyceride (TG) levels ($p < 5 \times 10^{-8}$). In the UK-Biobank (UKBB) GWAS dataset for self-reported high-cholesterol and in the Million Veteran Program (MVP) GWAS dataset for plasma TC, LDL-cholesterol, HDL-cholesterol, and TG, the prostasin association with the plasma lipid traits was replicated ($p < 5 \times 10^{-8}$). A detailed mechanistic investigation on prostasin's functional role in cholesterol and lipid metabolism should soon be on the horizon.

References

1. Yu JX, Chao L, Chao J (1995). Molecular cloning, tissue-specific expression, and cellular localization of human prostasin mRNA. *J Biol Chem.* 270(22):13483–13489.
2. Yu JX, Chao L, Chao J (1994). Prostasin is a novel human serine proteinase from seminal fluid. Purification, tissue distribution, and localization in prostate gland. *J Biol Chem.* 269(29):18843–18848.
3. Khandekar G, Iyer N, Jagadeeswaran P (2020). Prostasin and hepatocyte growth factor B in factor VIIa generation: Serine protease knockdowns in zebrafish. *Res Pract Thromb Haemost.* 4(7):1150–1157.
4. Sundaramoorthi H, Khandekar G, Kim S, Jagadeeswaran P (2015). Knockdown of αIIb by RNA degradation by delivering deoxyoligonucleotides piggybacked with control vivo-morpholinos into zebrafish thrombocytes. *Blood Cells Mol Dis.* 54(1):78–83.
5. https://www.gene-tools.com/vivomorpholinos
6. Kretz CA, Weyand AC, Shavit JA (2015). Modeling disorders of blood coagulation in the zebrafish. *Curr Pathobiol Rep.* 3(2):155–161.
7. Savoia A, Del Vecchio M, Totaro A, Perrotta S, Amendola G, Moretti A, Zelante L, Iolascon A (1999). An autosomal dominant thrombocytopenia gene maps to chromosomal region 10p. *Am J Hum Genet.* 65(5):1401–1405.
8. Johnson HJ, Gandhi MJ, Shafizadeh E, Langer NB, Pierce EL, Paw BH, Gilligan DM, Drachman JG (2009). In vivo inactivation of MASTL kinase results in thrombocytopenia. *Exp Hematol.* 37(8):901–908.
9. Mok SC, Chao J, Skates S, Wong K, Yiu GK, Muto MG, Berkowitz RS, Cramer DW (2001). Prostasin, a potential serum marker for ovarian cancer: identification through microarray technology. *J Natl Cancer Inst.* 93(19):1458–1464.
10. Bernardi F, Mariani G (2021). Biochemical, molecular and clinical aspects of coagulation factor VII and its role in hemostasis and thrombosis. *Haematologica.* 106(2):351–362.

11. Krishnamachary B, Cook C, Kumar A, Spikes L, Chalise P, Dhillon NK (2021). Extracellular vesicle-mediated endothelial apoptosis and EV-associated proteins correlate with COVID-19 disease severity. *J Extracell Vesicles.* 10(9):e12117.
12. Balbi C, Burrello J, Bolis S, Lazzarini E, Biemmi V, Pianezzi E, Burrello A, Caporali E, Grazioli LG, Martinetti G, Fusi-Schmidhauser T, Vassalli G, Melli G, Barile L (2021). Circulating extracellular vesicles are endowed with enhanced procoagulant activity in SARS-CoV-2 infection. *EBioMedicine.* 67:103369.
13. Grover SP, Mackman N (2018). Tissue factor: An essential mediator of hemostasis and trigger of thrombosis. *Arterioscler Thromb Vasc Biol.* 38(4):709–725.
14. van der Lubbe N, Jansen PM, Salih M, Fenton RA, van den Meiracker AH, Danser AH, Zietse R, Hoorn EJ (2012). The phosphorylated sodium chloride cotransporter in urinary exosomes is superior to prostasin as a marker for aldosteronism. *Hypertension.* 60(3):741–748.
15. Olivieri O, Chiecchi L, Pizzolo F, Castagna A, Raffaelli R, Gunasekaran M, Guarini P, Consoli L, Salvagno G, Kitamura K (2013). Urinary prostasin in normotensive individuals: Correlation with the aldosterone to renin ratio and urinary sodium. *Hypertens Res.* 36(6):528–533.
16. Chen LM, Chai JC, Liu B, Strutt TM, McKinstry KK, Chai KX (2021). Prostasin regulates PD-L1 expression in human lung cancer cells. *Biosci Rep.* 41(7):BSR20211370.
17. Hummler E, Dousse A, Rieder A, Stehle JC, Rubera I, Osterheld MC, Beermann F, Frateschi S, Charles RP (2013). The channel-activating protease CAP1/Prss8 is required for placental labyrinth maturation. *PLoS One.* 8(2):e55796.
18. Erlich J, Parry GC, Fearns C, Muller M, Carmeliet P, Luther T, Mackman N (1999). Tissue factor is required for uterine hemostasis and maintenance of the placental labyrinth during gestation. *Proc Natl Acad Sci USA.* 96(14):8138–8143.
19. Mackman N (2004). Role of tissue factor in hemostasis, thrombosis, and vascular development. *Arterioscler Thromb Vasc Biol.* 24(6):1015–1022.
20. https://www.gtexportal.org/home/gene/ENSG00000052344
21. List K, Hobson JP, Molinolo A, Bugge TH (2007). Co-localization of the channel activating protease prostasin/(CAP1/PRSS8) with its candidate activator, matriptase. *J Cell Physiol.* 213(1):237–245.

22. Chen LM, Skinner ML, Kauffman SW, Chao J, Chao L, Thaler CD, Chai KX (2001). Prostasin is a glycosylphosphatidylinositol-anchored active serine protease. *J Biol Chem.* 276(24):21434–21442.

23. Uchimura K, Hayata M, Mizumoto T, Miyasato Y, Kakizoe Y, Morinaga J, Onoue T, Yamazoe R, Ueda M, Adachi M, Miyoshi T, Shiraishi N, Ogawa W, Fukuda K, Kondo T, Matsumura T, Araki E, Tomita K, Kitamura K (2014). The serine protease prostasin regulates hepatic insulin sensitivity by modulating TLR4 signalling. *Nat Commun.* 5:3428.

24. Sekine T, Takizawa S, Uchimura K, Miyazaki A, Tsuchiya K (2021). Liver-specific overexpression of prostasin attenuates high-fat diet-induced metabolic dysregulation in mice. *Int J Mol Sci.* 22(15):8314.

25. Chen M, Chen LM, Chai KX (2006). Androgen regulation of prostasin gene expression is mediated by sterol-regulatory element-binding proteins and SLUG. *Prostate.* 66(9):911–920.

26. Su AI, Wiltshire T, Batalov S, Lapp H, Ching KA, Block D, Zhang J, Soden R, Hayakawa M, Kreiman G, Cooke MP, Walker JR, Hogenesch JB (2004). A gene atlas of the mouse and human protein-encoding transcriptomes. *Proc Natl Acad Sci USA.* 101(16):6062–6067.

27. Li Z, Votava JA, Zajac GJM, Nguyen JN, Leyva Jaimes FB, Ly SM, Brinkman JA, De Giorgi M, Kaul S, Green CL, St Clair SL, Belisle SL, Rios JM, Nelson DW, Sorci-Thomas MG, Lagor WR, Lamming DW, Eric Yen CL, Parks BW (2020). Integrating mouse and human genetic data to move beyond GWAS and identify causal genes in cholesterol metabolism. *Cell Metab.* 31(4):741–754.e5.

Chapter 14

Prostasin in Cancer

What is cancer? The National Cancer Institute has the following definition of cancer: "Cancer is a disease in which some of the body's cells grow uncontrollably and spread to other parts of the body". Cancers are grouped into six major categories based on the histological type, according to the International Classification of Diseases for Oncology[1]. They are carcinoma, sarcoma, myeloma, leukemia, lymphoma, and mixed types. Carcinomas originate from the epithelial tissues and account for 80–90% of all cancer cases. The epithelium is the body's surface covering the entire externally exposed parts of the body and topologically the lining of the internal organs, body cavities, and hollow organs. The secretory glands are also lined by epithelial cells which topologically are directly connected to the outside of the body via the ducts, also lined by epithelial cells.

The foremost function of the epithelium is the protection of the underlying tissues and cells from external insults, physical or material such as pathogens or chemicals. The epithelium, more precisely the epithelial cells, have multiple mechanisms to effectively protect our body in an active manner, and more important, to promote interactions and exchanges with the outside environment. The functions of the epithelium include secretion, absorption, filtration, diffusion, as well as sensory reception.

Not all epithelia are constructed the same way in different parts of the body and their functional requirements are very different. In the simple epithelium such as that in the kidney tubules and colon, there is only one layer of epithelial cells, while a stratified epithelium such as that in the skin and bladder consists of more than one layer of cells.

A pseudostratified epithelium such as that in the respiratory tract has just one layer of cells though they appear to be in layers. An epithelium can also be described by the cell shape, which is directly related to the function and moulded by the molecular landscape. There are squamous, cuboidal, and columnar epithelial cells. Depending on the specialization of the epithelium, the cells can be keratinized like the outermost layer of our skin, a stratified epithelium. Keratinized epithelial cells are anuclear and devoid of the cytoplasm but rich in the keratin proteins. The outermost layer of the oral cavity and the upper esophagus are parakeratinized and nucleated but also rich in keratins. The urinary bladder epithelial cells, also known as the urothelial cells, are transitional due to the organ's need to stretch, with the cells appearing as stratified cuboidal when relaxed but stratified squamous when distended.

The formation of an active epithelium barrier of our body is marked by the proper establishment of the cell-cell contacts and the signature junctions via the junctional proteins. This is not only essential in the formation of a nascent epithelium but also in wound healing, which prompted the concept of "contact inhibition". Such is the idea that the cells use the intercellular communications via the protein molecules, transmembrane and intracellular, to sense that the contact is complete and the cells are of the right types. It is this process that underlies the cancer definition of the NCI: When cells grow old or become damaged, they die, and new cells take their place. Sometimes this orderly process breaks down and abnormal or damaged cells grow and multiply when they shouldn't.

Prostasin is expressed in all epithelia. In humans, the most abundant source of prostasin in a bodily fluid is the seminal plasma (~8.6 μg/ml), wherein prostasin exists either in the free form[2] or a GPI-anchored membrane form[3] on the prostasomes, extracellular vesicles known as the exosomes but herein specifically from the prostate [Chen, unpublished results, University of Central Florida (UCF), USA]. In tissues, the prostate ranks the highest in prostasin expression, at ~25–50-fold higher than other tissues, such as the bronchi, colon, and kidney. The association of the prostasin expression change with cancers in an epithelium was first observed in the prostate and the breast, followed by other prostasin-expressing tissues.

14.1 Prostate and breast cancers

In 2001, Chen and colleagues[4] investigated prostasin expression in prostate cancer patient specimens. Prostasin was found to be down-regulated in advanced prostate cancers. Immunohistochemical analysis using polyclonal antibodies against the human prostasin[3] revealed that the prostasin protein is expressed in normal prostate epithelial cells, mostly at the apical surface towards the lumen and in prostatic secretions in the lumen, consistent with previous findings[2]. However, prostasin was less in quantity in low-grade prostate cancer specimens and sparsely present in high-grade prostate cancer specimens. *In vitro* cell line data corroborated the down-regulated expression of prostasin in prostate cancer, at both the mRNA and the protein levels, which could be detected in primary-cultured prostate epithelial cells (CC-2555, Lonza), in non-invasive human prostate cancer cells (LNCaP, ATCC), but barely detected in the invasive human prostate cancer cells (DU-145 and PC-3, ATCC). A forced over-expression of a recombinant human prostasin in the DU-145 and PC-3 cells reduces the cells' invasiveness. Furthermore, invasive prostate cancer cells derived from the transgenic adenocarcinoma of the mouse prostate (TRAMP) model[5] also have much less prostasin mRNA expression than the normal mouse prostate cells.

The reason to inspect the prostate specimens for prostasin expression *in situ* was not a difficult one because it is after all its namesake, but the findings were no less significant. The findings documented an association of prostasin expression change with a disease state, cancer of the prostate epithelial cells. Prostasin expression is abundant in the normal tissue and decreased to absence with the loss of the proper tissue architecture, as measured by the pathological grading of the cancer specimens. Moreover, the re-expression of prostasin in the invasive prostate cancer cell lines inhibited invasion, suggesting a potential mechanistic role for prostasin in maintaining the tissue architecture. Before this could be speculated further on behalf of prostasin, it needed to be shown that such is the case in other epithelial tissues.

Reduced prostasin expression was then observed in human breast cancer cells in 2002 by the same research group[6]. Prostasin expression at both the mRNA and the protein levels could readily be detected in normal human mammary epithelial cells (CC-2551, Lonza) and in non-invasive and non-metastatic breast carcinoma cell lines (MCF-7, MDA-MB-453, ATCC), but absent in highly invasive and metastatic breast carcinoma cell lines (MDA-MB-231 and MDA-MB-435s, ATCC). Similar to the phenotype observed in the invasive human prostate cancer cells upon prostasin re-expression, the invasiveness of human breast cancer cells MDA-MB-231 and MDA-MB-435s was reduced when prostasin was forcedly over-expressed in these cells. In either the prostate or the breast cancer cells re-expression of prostasin had no effect on cell proliferation *in vitro*.

The anti-invasion phenotype observed from the prostasin re-expression experiments does not necessarily suggest that the loss of prostasin in the invasive and metastatic cancer cells is mechanistic and causal. To begin addressing the molecular mechanisms, the prostasin down-regulation was investigated at the genomic DNA level in the cancer cell lines. To determine if there are structural mutations or rearrangements such as chromosomal translocations at the prostasin locus in the invasive cancer cell lines, an analysis of restriction fragment length polymorphism (RFLP) was performed using the genomic DNA of these cell lines. No evidence of gene loss or gross rearrangement was noted in the prostasin gene locus in the invasive breast cancer cell lines (Chai, unpublished results, UCF).

DNA methylation changes as a mechanism of gene expression regulation are critical to mammalian development, e.g., genomic imprinting and X-chromosome inactivation, but are also involved in the progression of cancers[7]. The addition of a methyl group on the cytosine residues in CpG dinucleotides in the regulatory regions of genes, along with the associated histone modifications, could repress the gene transcription by inducing chromatin structure changes. Epigenetic silencing, i.e., without DNA sequence changes, is an alternative mechanism of loss of tumor suppressor gene expression and was amended to the Knudson two-hit hypothesis[8].

The prostasin gene promoter sequence (GenBank accession number U33446) was inspected. A region that encompasses the promoter and exon I from −1,048 to +228 was found to contain 28 CpG dinucleotides, with 19 clustering in a GC-rich domain but falling short of a true CpG-island. This region is defined by two restriction endonucleases Xho I and BamH I, yielding a genomic DNA fragment readily analysed by Southern blot hybridization.

The first epigenetic changes in the prostasin gene[6] in cancer cells were reported using a now obsolete technique known as "methylation-sensitive RFLP" involving methylation-sensitive restriction endonucleases, which cut at sites with unmethylated CpG dinucleotides. The restriction fragment patterns were then compared to those generated with a restriction enzyme that cut the same sites, methylated or not, to determine the methylation state of the CpG therein. Alternatively, the patterns cut by the methylation-sensitive enzymes alone across the different cell lines could be compared to deduce the CpG methylation information. The results indicated that the methylation state in this region correlates with the prostasin expression down-regulation in invasive breast cancer cells. Especially, methylation at the –96 site close to the transcription initiation site and/or in +24 site in the exon 1 non-coding region had more effects on the prostasin gene transcription. Demethylation, coupled with histone deacetylase (HDAC) inhibition, rescued the prostasin expression in the invasive breast cancer cells. The prostasin promoter methylation is also the mechanism of prostasin expression silencing in invasive prostate cancer cells, with induction of expression by demethylation and HDAC inhibition[9]. Demethylation-induced prostasin expression has also been reported in cells of gastric cancer[10], bladder cancer[11], and esophageal squamous cell carcinoma[12].

The growth and development of the prostate are regulated by androgens, while androgen blockade is often used to treat prostate cancer[13]. However, hormone-independent growth of prostate tumors can lead to fast tumor progression and metastasis. In 2003, Takahashi and colleagues[14] reported that prostasin expression was down-regulated in high-grade or hormone-refractory human prostate cancers (HRPC), suggesting that a hormonal regulation may contribute to the repressed prostasin expression in cancers. Treating the androgen-responsive human prostate cancer cell line LNCaP with up to 100 nM of dihydrotestosterone (DHT) did not affect the prostasin mRNA expression whereas this and much lower doses (1 nM) of DHT markedly induced the prostate-specific antigen (PSA) mRNA[15]. A lack of an apparent androgen-responsive element (ARE) in the prostasin gene promoter region prompted the search for intermediate factors that may play a role in the androgen response of prostasin expression in the prostate cells.

In 2006, Chen and colleagues[15] showed that androgen could affect prostasin gene expression via pathways involving the sterol-regulatory element-binding proteins (SREBPs) or the zinc-finger transcription factor Slug, both were up-regulated by DHT in the androgen-responsive LNCaP human prostate cancer cells. The independent and coordinate effects of the SREBPs and Slug on prostasin expression were investigated using the HEK293 normal human embryonic kidney cell line. A prostasin promoter-reporter gene construct was used in co-transfection experiments with plasmids containing the cDNA coding for the SREBPs or Slug. Independently, the prostasin promoter activity is up-regulated by SREBP1c and SREBP2 but repressed by Slug. When the prostasin promoter-reporter was co-transfected with both SREBP2 and Slug in varying ratios to simulate the coordinate overall effect of a DHT response in the prostate cells, the activation of the prostasin promoter by SREBP2 was dose-dependently reverted by Slug. This would suggest that prostasin expression in the LNCaP cells is dictated by the relative amounts of SREBP2 and Slug present in the cells and in response to androgen.

Not surprisingly, several sterol regulatory elements (SREs) are present in the prostasin gene, as reported by the same research group in 2006[16]. The SRE+98 site was identified as a novel and the major regulatory site along with others, including SRE-897, SRE-538, SRE+8, and SRE+71. A candidate E-box where Slug would bind[17,18] and repress prostasin expression is present at position −574. Slug expression is up-regulated in many cancers including prostate cancer[19]. It is possible that in the hormone-refractory prostate cancers, androgen receptor (AR) could be activated in an androgen-independent manner leading to a sustained up-regulation of Slug expression, repressing the prostasin expression.

Collectively, the molecular mechanism for prostasin expression down-regulation in the invasive and metastatic cancers may be attributed to a hypermethylation of the prostasin promoter, an up-regulation of transcription repressors such as Snail and Slug, and a down-regulation of transcription activators such as the SREBPs'. In addition, Bonnet and colleagues[20] in 2010 developed a module network interface algorithm based on probabilistic optimization techniques and showed that prostasin expression can be up-regulated by miRNA-200, but down-regulated by zinc finger E-box-binding homeobox 1 (Zeb1).

14.2 Bladder cancers

The Snail family of zinc-finger transcription factors, including Snail and Slug, are major players in the regulation of the epithelial-to-mesenchymal transition (EMT) during embryogenesis, tissue regeneration, or cancer metastasis[21]. A key target gene downstream of the Snail family transcription factors is the *CDH1* encoding E-cadherin. E-cadherin is an adhesive protein which forms homophilic binding at the cell surface holding cells together in the adherens junctions (AJs)[22]. In this regard, E-cadherin is a tumour suppressor because a loss of its expression is associated with the EMT manifested by cell-cell dissociation and an increased cell migration potential. The regulation of E-cadherin expression and cell surface distribution by the Snail family transcription factors and Twist1 has a fate-determination role in early embryonic development during invagination. The alteration of the E-cadherin quantity and distribution on the surface of the embryo leads to a mechanical tension that drives the invagination. Cancer is often referred to as "embryonic reawakening" and the early embryonic genes such as the Snail and Twist1 are commonly expressed or reawakened in cancers.

In vitro EMT was first introduced and described by Greenburg and Hay[23] in 1982 when they discovered that the adult lens epithelium and the embryonic epithelium lose their polarities and acquire mesenchyme morphology when cultured in collagen gel. These epithelial cells dissociate themselves from the tissue explant and migrate as individual cells inside and surrounding the collagen gel. This was the first description that the *in vitro* environment can induce well-differentiated epithelial cells to change shape and polarity, and to gain migration and invasion potential. Greenburg and Hay described this progression as the epithelial-to-mesenchymal transition and attributed the initiation of this transition to the alteration of the apical-membrane components by collagen. Perhaps collagen, an extracellular matrix component, triggered apical signalling pathways that would not have been initiated otherwise if the cells were kept *in vivo* and polarized. The activated apical surface became the leading end of a mesenchymal cell migrating inside the collagen gel. In this context, prostasin may have a function to maintain the apical membrane components in a conformation with the epithelial morphology. Such a function would be expected to have an interface with maintaining the presence of the E-cadherin protein and repressing the presence of Slug in the epithelial cells. All findings to date associate prostasin expression and function with the terminally differentiated epithelium. An altered expression of prostasin may affect epithelial cell differentiation conferring them with partial mesenchymal features such as proliferation and migration, a phenotype later reported by Bao and colleagues in 2019 in a mouse model in which *Prss8* was knocked-out in the gastrointestinal tract[24].

In 2009, Chen and colleagues[11] surveyed prostasin expression in a bladder cancer tissue microarray (TMA, ARY-HH0087) by means of immunochemistry. A panel of 16 urothelial and transitional cell carcinoma (TCC) cell lines were also evaluated. The results were similar to the expression patterns previously observed in the prostate and breast cancers or cell lines. The prostasin protein is present in the normal human urothelium, but less in high-grade TCC. Prostasin is expressed in a normal human urothelial cell line UROtsa but lost in many TCC cell lines. The loss of prostasin expression in the TCC cell lines is due to the hypermethylation of the prostasin promoter at the −96 CpG site. Demethylation or inhibition of histone deacetylase reactivated the prostasin promoter resulting in prostasin re-expression. Interestingly, the DNA methylation status of the UROsta cells is not changed upon a long-term treatment in culture with the cigarette smoke extract[25], while cigarette smoking is a well-known epidemiological risk factor of bladder cancer.

The most notable result in this study is that the loss of prostasin expression is correlated with the loss of E-cadherin expression and the loss of epithelial morphology, suggesting a regulatory role of prostasin on the EMT in bladder TCC cells. The precise mechanism by which prostasin regulates the EMT is not completely known, but a focus on E-cadherin and Slug is merited. A prostasin over-expression in the PC-3 prostate cancer cells up-regulates E-cadherin expression but down-regulates Slug expression[26], and this forced expression of prostasin in the PC-3 and DU-145 prostate cancer cells reduces the cells' invasiveness. Prostasin also up-regulates E-cadherin expression in the KU-7 cells[11]. In addition, a forced expression of prostasin in KU-7 greatly inhibited the anchorage-independent growth in soft agar. The KU-7 cells were studied as a model of bladder cancer by many research groups for a long time but were forensically typed to have been HeLa cells, including the specific lot used in the studies described above (Chai, unpublished results, UCF). The importance of the findings however, remains. Prostasin up-regulation of E-cadherin expression was also reported in other cancer cell lines, e.g., esophagus (KYSE450, EC9706)[12], liver (HCCLM3)[27], lung (A549)[28], colon (HCT116, SW480)[24], and oral squamous cell carcinoma (SAS, HSC-4)[29].

The up-regulation of E-cadherin by prostasin re-expression in the PC-3 human prostate cancer cells was not dependent on its serine protease activity because a protease-dead serine active-site variant (Ala) had a much more robust effect than the wild-type prostasin[26]. However, the down-regulation of the Slug mRNA was only observed with the wild-type prostasin, suggesting a protease-dependent mechanism. Clearly the Slug down-regulation could be a mechanism of E-cadherin up-regulation, which is well established. The robust E-cadherin up-regulation by the protease-dead prostasin variant is an *in vitro* artifact since this variant does not exist in nature. A potential alternative mechanism may be suggested from the concomitant robust up-regulation of matriptase by this unnatural variant. Matriptase was later shown to be co-expressed in human breast cancer cells with E-cadherin and are co-markers of breast epithelial differentiation and a mechanism against the EMT[30].

14.3 Ovarian cancer

Another pioneering research on the expression of prostasin in cancers was published in 2001 by Mok and colleagues[31], reporting that prostasin is up-regulated in ovarian cancers, as opposed to the state of being down-regulated in prostate and breast cancers. Immunoreactive prostasin was identified in normal ovarian tissues, but a stronger staining was observed in eight ovarian cancer specimens. It was presumed that the prostasin protein released from the ovarian cancer cells would end up in the patient bloodstream along the progression of cancer. Serum samples from 64 ovarian cancer patients and 137 non-ovarian cancer patients were screened for the presence of prostasin by means of enzyme-linked immunosorbent assay (ELISA). A higher prostasin level was evident in the sera of the ovarian cancer cases. After surgically removing the cancers, the serum prostasin level was reduced from the level before the surgery. The prostasin level was the highest in the sera of patients with stage II ovarian cancer, and thus, prostasin was suggested as a potential biomarker for early detection of ovarian cancer, which lacks means of early detection.

In 2009, Sun and colleagues[32] identified the zinc-finger protein 217 (*ZNF217*) as a key transcriptional regulator in ovarian cancer cells. They silenced the *ZNF217* gene in an ovarian cancer cell line HO-8910 and analysed the global gene expression profiles using an Affymetrix Gene Chip with the HG-U133 plus 2.0 arrays. With the aid of the Gene Ontology program, 164 genes were found to be down-regulated by at least 8-fold when compared to the levels in the non-silenced control cells. The prostasin gene was one of the 164 down-regulated genes.

In 2014, Yan and colleagues[33] showed that prostasin may regulate the CASP/PAK2-p34, MLCK/actin, JNK/c-Jun pathways, and render ovarian cancer cells sensitive to the chemotherapy drug paclitaxel. In this study, a reduced prostasin expression is shown to correlate with a high ERCC1 (excision repair cross-complementing 1) expression in ovarian cancers. A high ERCC1 expression level is associated with cancer cell chemoresistance. Over-expression of prostasin in the paclitaxel-resistant O432-RP ovarian cancer cells partially reversed their chemoresistance, resulting in smaller tumor masses in nude mice treated with paclitaxel. Interestingly, the over-expression of prostasin alone in the O432-RP cells could reduce the tumor size in the xenografts even before the paclitaxel treatment, with the O432-RP cells harboring the vector serving as the control.

In the same year, Ma and colleagues[34] from the same group identified the prostatic secretory protein 94 (PSP94, also named as microseminoprotein beta, MSMB) as an upstream regulatory protein for prostasin expression. Both PSP94 and prostasin were up-regulated in ovarian cancers of all stages. It should be mentioned, and as the authors indicated in their study, that over-expressing prostasin in the O432-RP cells *in vitro* kills >99.99% cells upon drug selection in the attempt of establishing a stable prostasin-overexpressing subline. Only less than 0.01% of the transfected cells survived the drug selection. It is unclear if the cells from the 1/10,000 of the O432-RP pool could still represent the parent O432-RP cells, especially in regard to cell proliferation, invasion, and metastasis, given that all cancer cells are heterogeneous in nature.

In our hands, we have had tried to over-express prostasin in a normal human bladder cell line (UROtsa) but without success. We had similar experiences that a majority of the UROtsa cells were dead after prostasin transfection and upon drug selection. It did not appear that the massive cell death was all caused by the antibiotic used for selection, as cells transfected with the vector survived and did not show this phenotype during the antibiotic selection. In addition, transient transfection of prostasin cDNA in the UROtsa cells resulted in over-expression of prostasin in these cells (Chen, unpublished results, UCF). It does appear that in a cell-type specific manner, a prostasin over-expression may induce cell death in tissue-cultured cells, normal or cancerous. However, the physiological significance of this unique phenotype is unclear.

14.4 Colon cancer

In normal colorectal tissues, the prostasin protein is mainly localized on the apical plasma membrane as evaluated by immunohistochemistry. The prostasin mRNA expression as evaluated by reverse-transcription/quantitative polymerase chain reaction (RT-qPCR) is slightly but statistically significantly decreased in colorectal cancers (CRC) when compared to the normal tissues from the same individuals[35]. A lower expression of prostasin correlates with a low overall and disease-free survival time[36], but such a correlation was not noted in another study[37]. Over-expression of prostasin in the HCT116 CRC cells reduces tumor growth and metastasis of xenografts in nude mice, possibly involving the down-regulation of the Sphk1/S1p/Stat3/Akt signaling pathway. In addition, colon epithelial-specific silencing of prostasin expression in transgenic mice (*Prss8^{fl/fl}*, *p-Villin-Cre⁺*) results in spontaneous tumorigenesis in the colon[24]. This was the first study to describe that without prostasin expression in the colon epithelium, the epithelial cells proliferate at a higher rate and migrate faster. This phenotype indicates that the prostasin-deficient epithelial cells are less differentiated and possess mesenchymal cell characteristics. Bao and colleagues suggested that the Wnt/β-catenin, EMT, and stem cell signaling pathways are involved in the spontaneous tumor development and progression in the colon. Interestingly, in a similar intestine-specific prostasin knockout mouse model *Prss8^{KO}* (*Prss8^{lox/Δ}*; *villin::Cre^{tg/0}*, generated by mating the *Prss8^{Δ/+}*;*villin::Cre^{tg/0}* mice with the *Prss8^{lox/lox}* mice), the prostasin-deficient mouse colon had a normal gross anatomy in terms of the length-to-body weight ratio and a normal histology including the number of crypt cells which house the stem cells, and are capable of regenerating all intestinal cell types. The intestinal permeability was not compromised, indicating that an absence of prostasin alone does not affect the normal intestinal barrier function in mice. However, without prostasin, the ENaC activity in the colon was limited when the mice were fed with regular or low salt diet[38]. A speculative explanation of this discrepancy in the colon prostasin KO models is the difference in age of the animals used. The mice used for the cancer study were aged 12–36 weeks, while that for the ENaC activity study were aged 6–12 weeks. In addition, it is not clear if genetic backgrounds of the mice used in the two studies were contributing factors to the phenotypes. Further, in the mouse model (*Prss8^{ΔIEC}*) created by Sugitani and colleagues[39] in 2020, colonic epithelial cells did not show abnormal histology within the first 6–8 weeks without the prostasin expression. Again, age may be a factor among all other possible reasons.

14.5 Gastric and cervical cancers

In 2008, Sakashita and colleagues[10] analyzed 108 gastric cancer tumor specimens. The total RNA was extracted from the tumors and the normal mucosa. By means of RT-qPCR, the prostasin mRNA expression was found to be lower in the tumor samples. Accordingly, the immunoreactive prostasin protein was less in the tumors as well. It was suggested that the down-regulation of prostasin expression in gastric tumors is due to DNA hypermethylation because prostasin expression was reactivated in gastric cancer cell lines MKN1 and AZ521 after a demethylation treatment. In addition, a short survival time was associated with the lower prostasin expression in gastric cancer patients.

An alternative mechanism for down-regulating prostasin expression in gastric cancers was suggested by Sun *et al.* in 2016[40], where prostasin may be silenced by the antisense-transcribed long-non-coding RNA (lncRNA) HOXA11-AS. HOXA11-AS is specifically up-regulated in gastric cancers and the up-regulation is correlated with gastric cancer progression and poor prognosis. RNA-sequencing (RNA-seq) analysis identified prostasin as a downstream target of HOXA11-AS. Knocking down HOXA11-AS in gastric cancer cells BGC823, SGC7901, and MGC803 up-regulated prostasin expression, possibly via down-regulating the EZH2 (enhancer of zeste homology 2, a histone-lysine N-methyltransferase enzyme) and LSD1 (lysine-specific histone demethylase 1A) expression because silencing EZH2 or LSD1 increased prostasin mRNA expression. Further analysis by means of Chromatin Immunoprecipitation (ChIP) assay indicated that both EZH2 and LSD1 could bind to the *PRSS8* promoter at the −1264 location. The binding mediates methylation of the H3 histone protein to tri-methylated at Lys27 (H3K27me3) and di-methylated at Lys4 (H3K4me2). Silencing HOXA11-AS could reduce the binding of EZH2 and LSD1 to the *PRSS8* promoter thus increasing prostasin expression.

Another example of lncRNA inhibiting prostasin expression is LINP1 (long-non-coding RNA in non-homologous end joining (NHEJ) pathway 1), which is significantly up-regulated in cervical cancer (CC) tumors when compared to the adjacent normal tissues. Silencing LINP1 in CC cells Caski and C33A up-regulated prostasin expression. Similar to HOXA11-AS, LINP1 is possibly serving as a scaffold involving EZH2 and LSD1, as well as DNMT1 (DNA methyltransferase 1) in the regulation of prostasin gene expression[41].

A recent study by Zhu and colleagues[42] in 2022 suggested a miR-146b-3p binding site in the 3′-UTR (untranslated region) of the PRSS8 mRNA, mapped by using the Targetscan software. They further confirmed that an over-expression of miR-146b-3p down-regulates PRSS8 expression in the HCT116 and SW620 colon cancer cells, while an increased expression of PRSS8 was observed in cells with over-expression of lncRNA LINC00893 (Long intergenic non-protein coding RNA 893), which is a binding partner for miR-146b-3p as predicted by the bioinformatics tool LncBase V2. It is possible that LINC00893 binds to miR-146b-3p, depleting the binding potential of miR-146b-3p to PRSS8 to maintain the PRSS8 expression at a higher level. On one hand, LINC00893 has been shown to have anti-tumor properties, suppressing the growth, migration, and invasion of tumor cells, as well as inhibiting the epithelial-mesenchymal transition. On the other hand, miR-146b-3p increases tumor growth and metastases.

14.6 Liver cancer

In 2016, Zhang and colleagues[27] analyzed 106 surgically removed hepatocellular carcinoma (HCC) tumors and found that the prostasin mRNA and protein levels were decreased in most HCC tumors (49.1%, 52/106) when compared to the matched adjacent non-tumor tissues. The low expression of prostasin is an independent prognostic factor for lower overall survival rates. Using HCC cell lines HCCLM3 (highly metastatic) and HepG2 (non-metastatic), it was shown that an over-expression of prostasin in the HCCLM3 cells inhibited cell proliferation and invasion but promoted apoptosis and inhibited tumor growth as xenografts in nude mice. Conversely, silencing prostasin expression in the HepG2 cells increased cell proliferation and invasion but inhibited apoptosis and promoted tumor growth as xenografts in nude mice. The proposed signaling pathways were up-regulated expression of PTEN, E-cadherin, and Bax in the HCCLM3 cells over-expressing prostasin, but up-regulated expression of Bcl-2, MMP9, and N-cadherin in the prostasin-silenced HepG2 cells.

In 2017, Ashida and colleagues[43] carried out a High-tech Omics-based Patient Evaluation (HOPE) project which utilized surgically resected tumor specimens from 92 cases of HCC. Gene expression profiling analysis was performed using the SurePrint G3 Human Gene Expression 8×60 K v2 Microarray (Agilent Technologies, Santa Clara, CA, USA) hybridized with fluorescence-labeled RNA from the 92 cases. The GeneSpring GX software (Agilent Technologies) and Microsoft Excel were used to analyze the data, and prostasin was identified as the top down-regulated gene (64%, 59/92) with at least a 10-fold change between the tumor and non-tumor tissues. However, prostasin was not identified as an independent prognosis factor.

14.7 Esophageal squamous cell carcinoma

In 2016, Bao and colleagues[12] reported prostasin expression down-regulation in esophageal squamous cell carcinoma (ESCC) with a possible mechanism of DNA hypermethylation both in the tumor tissues and in ESCC cell lines KYSE450 and EC9706. A home-made ESCC tissue microarray (TMA) from 362 cases obtained from a local tissue bank was analyzed by means of immunohistochemistry. Immunoreactive prostasin was less in the invasive cancers and the reduced prostasin is correlated with poor differentiation of the tumors and a shorter survival time of the patients. Demethylation treatment of the ESCC cells reactivated prostasin expression, inhibited cell proliferation, motility, and migration, and induced cell cycle arrest. In addition, the expression of p21 and E-cadherin was up-regulated and that of cyclin D1, Twist, and Snail was down-regulated along with the prostasin reactivation, suggesting that these molecules may be involved in an interactive network regulated by prostasin.

14.8 Lung cancer

In 2017, Ma and colleagues[28] reported that prostasin is expressed in the BEAS-2B normal human bronchial epithelial cell line but the expression level is reduced in several non-small cell lung cancer (NSCLC) cell lines including NCI-1993, PC-9, and A549. Over-expression of prostasin in the A549 cells inhibited cell growth, migration, and invasion *in vitro*, and tumor growth *in vivo* as xenografts in nude mice. Upon prostasin over-expression in the A549 cells, the E-cadherin expression was up-regulated, while the JAK/Stat3 signaling pathway was inhibited. It was suggested that prostasin in the A549 cells may have suppressed the EMT.

In 2021, Chen and colleagues[44] used the Calu-3 (ATCC) human lung adenocarcinoma cell line, another NSCLC cell line, and established several sublines including a prostasin knockout subline (Calu-3KO), a prostasin over-expression subline (Calu-3Pro), an active-site mutant prostasin over-expression subline (Calu-3ProM), and a GPI-anchor-free prostasin over-expression subline (Calu-3ProG). They then analyzed the IFNγ-induced programmed death-ligand 1 (PD-L1) expression in these sublines. It was shown that upon IFNγ stimulation, the PD-L1 expression was up-regulated in all sublines but more prominently in the Calu-3Pro subline. Potential signaling cross-talks between the IFNγ pathways and the epidermal growth factor-epidermal growth factor receptor (EGF-EGFR) pathway involving protein kinase C alpha (PKCα) and mitogen-activated protein kinase (MAPK) could be responsible for the regulation of the PD-L1 expression by prostasin serine protease. More important, exosomes isolated from the Calu-3Pro subline carry both active prostasin and PD-L1 on the exosome membranes. PD-L1 is a negative regulator in immune surveillance and is the target for the drug atezolizumab in cancer immunotherapy. How prostasin regulates the action of PD-L1 in tumor immune evasion or tumor response to antibody-based treatment remains to be elucidated.

14.9 Glioma

Prostasin is mainly expressed in the epithelial cells in humans, rarely in non-epithelial cells. In carcinomas, the prostasin expression is usually down-regulated in the high-grade cancers or the invasive, metastatic cancer cell lines, while over-expressing prostasin reduces the invasiveness and metastatic potential, or proliferation and tumor growth.

Glioma, a type of tumor originating from the glial cells, was investigated with a focus on the expression and function of prostasin by Yang and colleagues in 2017[45]. Among 20 glioma patient samples, prostasin expression at both the mRNA and the protein levels is ~50% less when compared with that in the normal brain samples matched with the glioma samples. Consistent with the data of glioma tissues, the prostasin expression is ~50% less in two glioma cell lines, T98G and HS683, when compared with that in normal human astrocytes (NHA). *In vitro*, over-expression of a recombinant prostasin in the T98G and HS683 glioma cells reduced cell proliferation, migration, and invasion possibly by suppressing the Akt/mTOR signaling pathway. *In vivo*, when injected subcutaneously into nude mice (female BALB/c), the T98G cells over-expressing prostasin had a reduced tumor growth in volume and weight when compared with the tumors from T98G cells without the prostasin over-expression.

Interestingly, as described at the ATCC (American Type Culture Collection, Manassas, VA, USA), both the T98G and HS683 cells are fibroblasts and non-tumorigenic, they do not produce tumors in nude mice. It is of interest whether the T98G and HS683 cell lines used by Yang and colleagues remained the same in properties and characteristics as described at the ATCC in regard to tumorigenicity. Nevertheless, as prostasin is known for its anti-invasion and anti-metastasis functions, it could be an alternative way of treating cancers if proven that an ectopic expression of prostasin in non-epithelial cancer cells reduces the aggressive cancer cell properties.

14.10 Oral squamous cell carcinoma (OSCC)

In 2021, Yamamoto and colleagues[29] analyzed 119 surgically resected OSCC tumors by means of immunohistochemistry. Immunoreactive prostasin was found to be less in the tumor tissues (63%, 75/119). OSCC tumors with a low prostasin level usually had a higher histological grade and appeared as a more infiltrative cancer cell morphology. A lower level of prostasin also correlated with a lower overall survival rate in patients after tumor resection. Over-expression of prostasin in OSCC cell lines SAS and HSC-4 suppressed cell proliferation, migration, and invasion, while silencing prostasin expression in the HSC-4 cells enhanced cell proliferation. Interestingly, in 2018, the same group[46] noted that a genetic deletion of hepatocyte growth factor activator inhibitor type-2 (HAI-2), a prostasin inhibitor, in the SAS and HSC-3 cells up-regulated prostasin expression. The up-regulated prostasin may be a contributing factor to the reduced invasiveness of these HAI-2-knockout cells.

14.11 Summary

The proteolytic activities of proteases are controlled by their natural and physiological inhibitors. In the microenvironment of normal tissues, a finely balanced expression and a well-controlled interaction among the inhibitors, proteases, and the substrates allow the normal physiological functions to go on.

A traditional view of proteases in cancer biology is that in the microenvironment of malignant tumor tissues, this balance is often tipped towards an increased protease activity. As a result, the extracellular matrix can be degraded and the cell-cell connections are lost, enabling the malignant cells to migrate and invade to surrounding tissues, and eventually metastasize to distant tissue sites[47]. Conversely, recent research points to the roles of proteases in suppression of tumor progression[48]. Prostasin is included as one example with good evidence in support (Figure 14-1).

The prostasin expression is generally down-regulated in advanced cancers and the down-regulation is correlated with cancer progression and poor prognosis. Forced prostasin re-expression in advanced cancer cells may be an intervention for slowing down the cancer progression with a possibility of a regression toward cellular re-differentiation, in principle. In reality, the potential of using prostasin as a therapeutic agent may be hindered by multiple factors. First, it remains difficult to deliver a protein agent to solid tumors systemically or via its gene in a viral vector. Second, the tumors that have gained the highest malignancy are undifferentiated and the cellular machinery required for restoring a

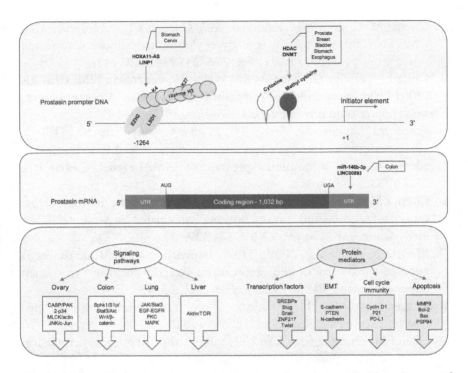

Figure 14-1. Summary of potential regulatory mechanisms and pathways of prostasin at the gene, the mRNA, and the protein levels.

differentiated state may have lost too many parts for a single molecular agent of prostasin to have very much of an effect. At least the emergence of exploiting the exosomes as a vehicle for delivery may offer the hope of overcoming the first obstacle. Herein lies the significance of the recent ascertainment of prostasin's presence in the exosomes in a fully functional capacity[44].

References

1. International Classification of Diseases for Oncology (Third Edition, ICD-O-3, https://training.seer.cancer.gov/icdo3/).
2. Yu JX, Chao L, Chao J (1994). Prostasin is a novel human serine proteinase from seminal fluid. Purification, tissue distribution, and localization in prostate gland. *J Biol Chem.* 269(29):18843–18848.

3. Chen LM, Skinner ML, Kauffman SW, Chao J, Chao L, Thaler CD, Chai KX (2001). Prostasin is a glycosylphosphatidylinositol-anchored active serine protease. *J Biol Chem.* 276(24):21434–21442.

4. Chen LM, Hodge GB, Guarda LA, Welch JL, Greenberg NM, Chai KX (2001). Down-regulation of prostasin serine protease: A potential invasion suppressor in prostate cancer. *Prostate.* 48(2):93–103.

5. Foster BA, Gingrich JR, Kwon ED, Madias C, Greenberg NM (1997). Characterization of prostatic epithelial cell lines derived from transgenic adenocarcinoma of the mouse prostate (TRAMP) model. *Cancer Res.* 57(16):3325–3330.

6. Chen LM, Chai KX (2002). Prostasin serine protease inhibits breast cancer invasiveness and is transcriptionally regulated by promoter DNA methylation. *Int J Cancer.* 97(3):323–329.

7. El-Osta A, Wolffe AP (2000). DNA methylation and histone deacetylation in the control of gene expression: Basic biochemistry to human development and disease. *Gene Expr.* 9(1-2):63–75.

8. Knudson AG Jr (1971). Mutation and cancer: Statistical study of retinoblastoma. *Proc Natl Acad Sci USA.* 68(4):820–823.

9. Chen LM, Zhang X, Chai KX (2004). Regulation of prostasin expression and function in the prostate. *Prostate.* 59(1):1–12.

10. Sakashita K, Mimori K, Tanaka F, Tahara K, Inoue H, Sawada T, Ohira M, Hirakawa K, Mori M (2008). Clinical significance of low expression of Prostasin mRNA in human gastric cancer. *J Surg Oncol.* 98(7): 559–564.

11. Chen LM, Verity NJ, Chai KX (2009). Loss of prostasin (PRSS8) in human bladder transitional cell carcinoma cell lines is associated with epithelial-mesenchymal transition (EMT). *BMC Cancer.* 9:377.

12. Bao Y, Wang Q, Guo Y, Chen Z, Li K, Yang Y, Zhang H, Dong H, Shen K, Yang W (2016). PRSS8 methylation and its significance in esophageal squamous cell carcinoma. *Oncotarget.* 7(19):28540–28555. Erratum in: *Oncotarget.* 2017 May 2;8(18):30617–30618.

13. Cunha GR, Donjacour AA, Cooke PS, Mee S, Bigsby RM, Higgins SJ, Sugimura Y (1987). The endocrinology and developmental biology of the prostate. *Endocr Rev.* 8(3):338–362.

14. Takahashi S, Suzuki S, Inaguma S, Ikeda Y, Cho YM, Hayashi N, Inoue T, Sugimura Y, Nishiyama N, Fujita T, Chao J, Ushijima T, Shirai T (2003). Down-regulated expression of prostasin in high-grade or hormone-refractory human prostate cancers. *Prostate.* 54(3):187–193.

15. Chen M, Chen LM, Chai KX (2006). Androgen regulation of prostasin gene expression is mediated by sterol-regulatory element-binding proteins and SLUG. *Prostate*. 66(9):911–920.
16. Chen M, Chen LM, Chai KX (2006). Mechanisms of sterol regulatory element-binding protein-2 (SREBP-2) regulation of human prostasin gene expression. *Biochem Biophys Res Commun*. 346(4):1245–1253.
17. Batlle E, Sancho E, Franci C, Dominguez D, Monfar M, Baulida J, Garcia De Herreros A (2000). The transcription factor snail is a repressor of E-cadherin gene expression in epithelial tumour cells. *Nat Cell Biol*. 2:84–89.
18. Bolós V, Peinado H, Perez-Moreno MA, Fraga MF, Esteller M, Cano A (2003). The transcription factor Slug represses E-cadherin expression and induces epithelial to mesenchymal transitions: A comparison with Snail and E47 repressors. *J Cell Sci*. 116(Pt 3):499–511.
19. Alves CC, Carneiro F, Hoefler H, Becker KF (2009). Role of the epithelial-mesenchymal transition regulator Slug in primary human cancers. *Front. Biosci*. 14(8):3035–3050.
20. Bonnet E, Tatari M, Joshi A, Michoel T, Marchal K, Berx G, Van de Peer Y (2010). Module network inference from a cancer gene expression data set identifies microRNA regulated modules. *PLoS One*. 5(4):e10162.
21. Jolly MK, Ware KE, Gilja S, Somarelli JA, Levine H (2017). EMT and MET: Necessary or permissive for metastasis? *Mol Oncol*. 11(7):755–769.
22. Vendome J, Felsovalyi K, Song H, Yang Z, Jin X, Brasch J, Harrison OJ, Ahlsen G, Bahna F, Kaczynska A, Katsamba PS, Edmond D, Hubbell WL, Shapiro L, Honig B (2014). Structural and energetic determinants of adhesive binding specificity in type I cadherins. *Proc Natl Acad Sci USA*. 111(40):E4175–E4184.
23. Greenburg G, Hay ED (1982). Epithelia suspended in collagen gels can lose polarity and express characteristics of migrating mesenchymal cells. *J Cell Biol*. 95(1):333–339.
24. Bao Y, Guo Y, Yang Y, Wei X, Zhang S, Zhang Y, Li K, Yuan M, Guo D, Macias V, Zhu X, Zhang W, Yang W (2019). PRSS8 suppresses colorectal carcinogenesis and metastasis. *Oncogene*. 38(4):497–517. Erratum in: *Oncogene*. 2021 Mar;40(10):1922–1924.
25. Chen LM, Nergard JC, Ni L, Rosser CJ, Chai KX (2013). Long-term exposure to cigarette smoke extract induces hypomethylation at the RUNX3 and IGF2-H19 loci in immortalized human urothelial cells. *PLoS One*. 8(5):e65513.

26. Chen M, Fu YY, Lin CY, Chen LM, Chai KX (2007). Prostasin induces protease-dependent and independent molecular changes in the human prostate carcinoma cell line PC-3. *Biochim Biophys Acta.* 1773(7):1133–1140.

27. Zhang L, Jia G, Shi B, Ge G, Duan H, Yang Y (2016). PRSS8 is down-regulated and suppresses tumour growth and metastases in hepatocellular carcinoma. *Cell Physiol Biochem.* 40(3–4):757–769.

28. Ma C, Ma W, Zhou N, Chen N, An L, Zhang Y (2017). Protease serine S1 family member 8 (PRSS8) inhibits tumor growth in vitro and in vivo in human non-small cell lung cancer. *Oncol Res.* 25(5):781–787.

29. Yamamoto K, Yamashita F, Kawaguchi M, Izumi A, Kiwaki T, Kataoka H, Kaneuji T, Yamashita Y, Fukushima T (2021). Decreased prostasin expression is associated with aggressiveness of oral squamous cell carcinoma. *Hum Cell.* 34(5):1434–1445.

30. Zoratti GL, Tanabe LM, Hyland TE, Duhaime MJ, Colombo É, Leduc R, Marsault E, Johnson MD, Lin CY, Boerner J, Lang JE, List K (2016). Matriptase regulates c-Met mediated proliferation and invasion in inflammatory breast cancer. *Oncotarget.* 7(36):58162–58173.

31. Mok SC, Chao J, Skates S, Wong K, Yiu GK, Muto MG, Berkowitz RS, Cramer DW (2001). Prostasin, a potential serum marker for ovarian cancer: identification through microarray technology. *J Natl Cancer Inst.* 93(19):1458–1464.

32. Sun G, Qin J, Qiu Y, Gao Y, Yu Y, Deng Q, Zhong M (2009). Microarray analysis of gene expression in the ovarian cancer cell line HO-8910 with silencing of the ZNF217 gene. *Mol Med Rep.* 2(5):851–855.

33. Yan BX, Ma JX, Zhang J, Guo Y, Mueller MD, Remick SC, Yu JJ (2014). Prostasin may contribute to chemoresistance, repress cancer cells in ovarian cancer, and is involved in the signaling pathways of CASP/PAK2-p34/actin. 5(1):e995.

34. Ma JX, Yan BX, Zhang J, Jiang BH, Guo Y, Riedel H, Mueller MD, Remick SC, Yu JJ (2014). PSP94, an upstream signaling mediator of prostasin found highly elevated in ovarian cancer. *Cell Death Dis.* 5(9):e1407.

35. Selzer-Plon J, Bornholdt J, Friis S, Bisgaard HC, Lothe IM, Tveit KM, Kure EH, Vogel U, Vogel LK (2009). Expression of prostasin and its inhibitors during colorectal cancer carcinogenesis. *BMC Cancer.* 9:201.

36. Bao Y, Li K, Guo Y, Wang Q, Li Z, Yang Y, Chen Z, Wang J, Zhao W, Zhang H, Chen J, Dong H, Shen K, Diamond AM, Yang W (2016).

Tumor suppressor PRSS8 targets Sphk1/S1P/Stat3/Akt signaling in colorectal cancer. *Oncotarget.* 7(18):26780–26792.

37. Cavalieri D, Dolara P, Mini E, Luceri C, Castagnini C, Toti S, Maciag K, De Filippo C, Nobili S, Morganti M, Napoli C, Tonini G, Baccini M, Biggeri A, Tonelli F, Valanzano R, Orlando C, Gelmini S, Cianchi F, Messerini L, Luzzatto L (2007). Analysis of gene expression profiles reveals novel correlations with the clinical course of colorectal cancer. *Oncol Res.* 16(11):535–548.

38. Malsure S, Wang Q, Charles RP, Sergi C, Perrier R, Christensen BM, Maillard M, Rossier BC, Hummler E (2014). Colon-specific deletion of epithelial sodium channel causes sodium loss and aldosterone resistance. *J Am Soc Nephrol.* 25(7):1453–1464.

39. Sugitani Y, Nishida A, Inatomi O, Ohno M, Imai T, Kawahara M, Kitamura K, Andoh A (2020). Sodium absorption stimulator prostasin (PRSS8) has an anti-inflammatory effect via downregulation of TLR4 signaling in inflammatory bowel disease. *J Gastroenterol.* 55(4): 408–417.

40. Sun M, Nie F, Wang Y, Zhang Z, Hou J, He D, Xie M, Xu L, De W, Wang Z, Wang J (2016). LncRNA HOXA11-AS promotes proliferation and invasion of gastric cancer by scaffolding the chromatin modification factors PRC2, LSD1, and DNMT1. *Cancer Res.* 76(21):6299–6310.

41. Wu L, Gong Y, Yan T, Zhang H (2020). LINP1 promotes the progression of cervical cancer by scaffolding EZH2, LSD1, and DNMT1 to inhibit the expression of KLF2 and PRSS8. *Biochem Cell Biol.* 98(5):591–599.

42. Zhu J, Jiang C, Hui H, Sun Y, Tao M, Liu Y, Qian X (2022). Overexpressed lncRNA LINC00893 suppresses progression of colon cancer by binding with miR-146b-3p to upregulate PRSS8. *J Oncol.* 2022:8002318.

43. Ashida R, Okamura Y, Ohshima K, Kakuda Y, Uesaka K, Sugiura T, Ito T, Yamamoto Y, Sugino T, Urakami K, Kusuhara M, Yamaguchi K (2017). CYP3A4 gene is a novel biomarker for predicting a poor prognosis in hepatocellular carcinoma. *Cancer Genomics Proteomics.* 14(6):445–453.

44. Chen LM, Chai JC, Liu B, Strutt TM, McKinstry KK, Chai KX (2021). Prostasin regulates PD-L1 expression in human lung cancer cells. *Biosci Rep.* 41(7):BSR20211370.

45. Yang HY, Fang DZ, Ding LS, Hui XB, Liu D (2017). Overexpression of protease serine 8 inhibits glioma cell proliferation, migration, and invasion via suppressing the Akt/mTOR signaling pathway. *Oncol Res.* 25(6):923–930.

46. Yamamoto K, Kawaguchi M, Shimomura T, Izumi A, Konari K, Honda A, Lin C, Johnson MD, Yamashita Y, Fukushima T, Kataoka H (2018). Hepatocyte growth factor activator inhibitor type-2 (HAI-2)/SPINT2 contributes to invasive growth of oral squamous cell carcinoma cells. *Oncotarget.* 9(14):11691–11706.
47. Fischer A (1946). Mechanism of the proteolytic activity of malignant tissue cells. *Nature.* 157:442.
48. López-Otín C, Matrisian LM (2007). Emerging roles of proteases in tumour suppression. *Nat Rev Cancer.* 7(10):800–808.

Chapter 15

Prostasin Substrates, Regulators, and Inhibitors

15.1 A substrate or an inhibitor — synthetic

Almost 30 years after its discovery, the exact natural substrates, inhibitors, and regulators of prostasin are still in question. Meanwhile, just as with other trypsin-like serine proteases, prostasin has been shown to cleave synthetic peptide substrates for trypsin such as Boc-QAR-AMC or D-PFR-MCA, or to be inhibited by trypsin-like protease inhibitors such as benzamidine or phenylmethylsulfonyl fluoride (PMSF) in the *in vitro* setting.

A substrate of an enzyme can become an inhibitor of the enzyme if the substrate itself does not dissociate from the enzyme easily after the cleavage or undergoes a cleavage-induced conformational change preventing the enzyme from regaining the enzyme activity. In some cases, these types of inhibitors, synthetic or naturally occurring, are referred to as suicide inhibitors.

To explore for small molecule inhibitors of prostasin, in 2008, Tully and colleagues[1] used an optimized peptide substrate Ac-KHYR-acmc of prostasin as a template, replaced the labile coumarin amide with an electrophilic α-ketoheterocycle transition-state analog mimic to develop several potential synthetic peptidomimetic inhibitors. They reported that compound 23 is a potent reversible inhibitor of prostasin with a K_i of 0.012 μM.

The optimized peptide substrate Ac-KHYR-acmc was selected based on the result from a positional scanning of combinatorial substrate libraries[2]. It was postulated that the preferred peptide substrate for prostasin would have arginine (R) or lysine (K) in the P1 position, basic or large hydrophobic amino acids in P2, histidine (H), lysine or arginine in P3 and arginine or lysine in P4. The α-ketoheterocycle based inhibitors have been used often in the development of serine protease inhibitors, due to the reversibility of these transition-state analogs[3,4].

The effort of converting the substrate Ac-KHYR-acmc into an inhibitor by changing the labile coumarin amide to an α-ketoheterocycle transition-state analog did not endow much inhibitory activity. Guided by the X-ray structures of each compound bound to the active site of prostasin, changing amino acids, and adding various substituents to the amino acids of the peptides had led to the development of compound 23. The structure-activity relationship (SAR) analysis of the substituents on the P2 proline reveals that the S2 subsite of the prostasin protein prefers non-polar, hydrophobic moieties, especially the six-membered aliphatic rings. Therefore, the substituent *para*-chlorobenzylether moiety on the P2 proline allowed compound 23 to fit better in the prostasin active site pocket. The α-ketobenzoxazole substituent added to the P1 lysine sits in the oxyanion hole interacting with the active site of prostasin. The P3 amino acid is essential for maintaining the length of the peptide and functions better with D-hPhe (D-Homophenylalamine). The final peptidomimetic inhibitor has a sequence and structure of Cbz-D-hPhe-Pro(*para*-chlorobenzylether)-Lys-ketobenzoxazole, quite different from the initial optimized substrate Ac-KHYR-acmc.

Due to the small size and unique structure, the same amino acid residues of the small synthetic substrates or inhibitors may behave differently if they are in a naturally occurring physiological substrate or inhibitor of prostasin. For example, the Leu-Ile-Ala-Arg residues in the positions of P4–P1 in the human protease nexin-1 (PN-1) reactive site may be a good substrate of prostasin *in vitro* as a peptidomimetic substrate (Chen, unpublished results, UCF) but is actually a suicide inhibitor when present naturally in the entire PN-1 polypeptide. Interestingly, a perfect match of a predicated preferred cleavage site by prostasin, RRAR↓SVAS is seen in the extracellular domains of the epithelial sodium channel (ENaC) alpha-subunit at P4–P4' (UniProtKB — P37088, amino acids 201–208) and in the

SARS-CoV-2 spike protein S1–S2 junction at 682–689 (UniProtKB — P0DTC2).

15.2 The epithelial sodium channel (ENaC)

Currently, the physiological substrates of human prostasin are unknown, but several potential candidates have been recognized and studied using *in vitro* cell lines and *in vivo* animal models.

The first and the best characterized potential naturally occurring substrate of prostasin is the epithelial sodium channel (ENaC). The ENaC with three subunits is located on the apical surface of the cell plasma membrane and functions as a sensor of Na^+ concentration in the extracellular environment. The ENaC activity can be regulated via a "feedback inhibition" relating to an increased intracellular Na^+ concentration and a decreased ENaC activity and/or density on the cell surface. A "self-inhibition" of ENaC activity occurs seconds after an increase of the extracellular Na^+, with Na^+ binding to the ENaC, leading to a reduction of the ENaC open probability to control the Na^+ entry into the cell[5-8]. The ENaC is activated by various but specific proteases during the biosynthesis inside the cell and on the surface of the plasma membrane. The latter is a mechanism of acquiring higher open probability of the Na^+ channel in response to higher demands. Prostasin is identified among others as an ENaC cleaving and activating enzyme on the apical plasma membrane both *in vitro* and *in vivo*.

In the kidney, the ENaC is expressed in the aldosterone-sensitive distal nephron where it regulates the reabsorption of Na^+, and in exchange, facilities K^+ secretion which is a fine-tuning step of the Na^+ absorption. Osmotically, water flows with the Na^+ into the cell when the ENaC is in action, regulating the extracellular volume and the blood pressure. Prostasin is co-localized with the ENaC in the distal nephron, but also found in the aldosterone-insensitive tubules in the kidney. The ENaC activity in the kidney is subjected to at least two layers of regulation, by aldosterone and/or prostasin.

In the lung, the ENaC is expressed in the airway and alveolar epithelial cells which are not sensitive to aldosterone regulation. Whereas prostasin plays key roles on the function of the ENaC to regulate the airway surface liquid (ASL), its own expression is regulated upon the ASL volume change.

In the colon of Sprague-Dawley rats fed with a low sodium diet or infused with aldosterone, prostasin expression is induced in the left colon or distal colon which is sensitive to aldosterone regulation. Coinciding with this, the ENaC expression is also increased.

In the skin, the functional relationship of prostasin and the ENaC may be dissociated as the ENaC is active in a skin-specific prostasin gene knockout animal model.

15.3 Receptor tyrosine kinases (RTK) and others

The initial characterization of the prostasin isolated from human seminal plasma suggested a preference of Arg-X as the peptide bond (the scissile bond) being cleaved in a substrate. This information and the prostasin's extracellular membrane anchorage prompted an investigation of the prototypic RTK, the epidermal growth factor receptor (EGFR, aka Her1/ErbB1) as a candidate substrate in the context of prostate biology and prostate cancer pathophysiology[9,10]. Investigating the RTKs as candidate prostasin substrates was further expanded to other members or subfamilies, such as Her-2, Her-3, and Her-4, as well as the insulin receptor (INSR), insulin-like growth factor I receptor (IGF-1R), platelet-derived growth factor receptors (PDGFRs) α and β, and never growth factor receptor A (TrkA)[11]. Prostasin was shown to be only weakly active toward Her-3 and PDGFRα, but not able to cleave other RTKs. These studies suggested that prostasin might have been involved in a protease cascade working in concert with other membrane-anchored serine proteases, such as matriptase, which is a proteolytic modifier of all the RTKs tested. A re-expression of prostasin in the PC-3 human prostate cancer cell line induced EGFR pathway signaling changes. Some of the prostasin re-expression phenotypes were also observed in the cells endowed with a protease-dead prostasin variant, suggesting a protease-independent mechanism[12]. The re-expression of the protease-dead prostasin variant was associated with a robust up-regulation of matriptase at the transcription level with a corresponding increase at the protein level. The molecular mechanism of the matriptase up-regulation remains unclear.

15.4 Protease-activated receptors (PARs)

There are four protease-activated receptors (PARs), known as PAR-1, PAR-2, PAR-3, and PAR-4, all belonging to the seven-transmembrane-domain G protein-coupled receptor (GPCR) super-family. The GPCR superfamily is massive, with greater than 800 human genes identified, representing approximately 4% of all the protein-coding genes. The PARs interact with proteases in the extracellular space and activate signaling pathways via the transmembrane domains serving as a hub to transmit signals from the outside in.

The PARs may be activated through several mechanisms[13]. The classical pathway is a direct proteolytic cleavage at the extracellular amino terminal region of the PARs, such as PAR-1, -3, -4 by thrombin or PAR-2 by trypsin. The cleaved small amino-terminal fragment is then used as the ligand to activate the PAR. Other mechanisms are dimerization of PARs at the cell membrane, post-translational modifi-cations via glycosylation, phosphorylation, or ubiquitination. In some cases, partnering with other receptors or cofactors can also regulate PAR activation, as well as cellular trafficking via degradation, recycling by endosomal, or compartmentalization.

In cell line studies, prostasin was suggested to down-regulate the PAR-2 activation pathway as assessed by cytokine expression down-stream of PAR-2[14]. Silencing the prostasin expression in the BPH-1 benign human prostate cell line up-regulated iNOS, while blocking the PAR-2 activation by a PAR-2 antagonist prevented the iNOS up-regulation in these cells, suggesting that prostasin may function to keep PAR-2 in a quiescent state. In addition, silencing prostasin also increased IL-6 and IL-8 mRNA expression, both are downstream effectors of PAR-2 activation.

In mice, prostasin is suggested to indirectly activate the PAR-2 singling pathways via activating matriptase which plays roles in neural tube closure[15]. Even when matriptase is in its zymogen form, PAR-2 can still be activated in the skin and colon, maintaining the normal developmental homeostasis of the epithelium, but not for hair follicle development[16]. It was suggested that prostasin, in this case, is the mediator in the PAR-2 activation. In another mouse model, the skin lesion and barrier dysfunction caused by an over-expression of prostasin can be diminished if the PAR-2 expression is knocked out at the same time, suggesting that PAR-2 is a downstream effector of prostasin[17].

15.5 Toll-like receptor 4 (TLR4)

TLR4 is a transmembrane protein expressed mainly in cells of the myeloid origin. It belongs to the pattern recognition receptor family. Lipopolysaccharide (LPS), a component of the outer membrane of Gram-negative bacteria, is the most well-known ligand recognized by TLR4. TLR4 initiated signaling pathways via activating NF-κB make TLR4 a master regulator of the inflammatory cytokine production in the activated innate immune system.

Prostasin may function to keep TLR4 silent in normal epithelial cells as it does in the case of PAR-2. Prostasin has been demonstrated in many studies to have anti-inflammatory functions using mouse models of bladder, liver, or colon inflammation[18–20]. The expression of prostasin and TLR4 is inversely correlated. In normal epithelial cells, prostasin is abundantly expressed while the TLR4 expression is hardly seen. When the prostasin expression is silenced genetically, the TLR4 expression is up-regulated, which dictates the downstream inflammatory cytokine production. Conversely, when the prostasin expression is genetically up-regulated in the inflamed tissues, the TLR4 expression is reduced and controlled at a low level.

15.6 The transmembrane protease, serine 13 (TMPRSS13)

TMPRSS13 is a splice variant of the mosaic serine protease large form (MSPL) in the hepsin/TMPRSS subfamily. TMPRSS13 is a type II single-pass transmembrane protein with the carboxyl terminal protease domain in the extracellular space.

The expression of prostasin and TMPRSS13 is also inversely correlated[21]. The TMPRSS13 mRNA is over-expressed in human breast cancers according to the Oncomine™ microarray database (TCGA breast dataset), but minimally expressed in the non-malignant human breast epithelial cell lines. Silencing the TMPRSS13 expression resulted in an increased prostasin expression in the HCC1937 human breast cancer cells. The molecular mechanism involves a TMPRSS13 cleavage of prostasin, removing the latter from the cells. In this sense, TMPRSS13 is a regulator of prostasin and prostasin is a substrate of TMPRSS13.

15.7 Matriptase — the beginning and the end of a cascade

Prostasin and matriptase are proposed to be a pair of enzyme-substrates in a proteolytic cascade in the epithelial cells[15,22], just as the coagulating serine protease cascade in the blood. Both enzymes in their zymogen forms can be used by the other one as a substrate to produce an activated enzyme which in turn could activate more zymogens. The activation reactions are reciprocal (Figure 15-1).

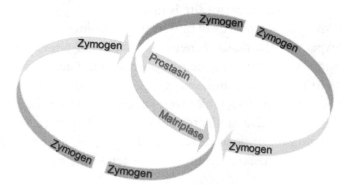

Figure 15-1. Prostasin and matriptase cleave and activate each other reciprocally. Yellow arrow: Active prostasin can convert matriptase zymogen to active matriptase (pink arrow), which can convert prostasin zymogen to active prostasin. Blue arrow: Prostasin zymogen can convert matriptase zymogen to active matriptase (pink arrow). Green arrow: Matriptase zymogen can convert prostasin zymogen to active prostasin (yellow arrow).

The functional dissociation of prostasin from matriptase is observed during the placenta formation in mice in the early stage of pregnancy. Prostasin is required to be present in the trophoblast cells which differentiate into a placenta but is not required in the embryoblasts which develop into an embryo[23]. Lacking the prostasin expression is embryonic lethal to mice, which cannot survive past E14.5. However, a matriptase gene knockout[24] does not prevent the embryos from developing to term, but the newborn mice survive only up to 48 hours due to skin defects that cause dehydration, leading to death. Prostasin as a stress sensor coordinate with matriptase to maintain the epithelial cells in the differentiated and functionally competent state.

In 2014, Peters and colleagues[25] generated a mouse model in which the prostasin active site was mutated from serine to alanine, i.e., *Prss8-S238A*, in the prostasin gene. This form of prostasin can be cleaved and activated to become a two-chain molecule, but the molecule itself does not possess any serine protease activity and cannot cleave other substrates such as matriptase.

In 2016, Friis and colleagues[26] generated a mouse model in which prostasin was kept as a single-chain zymogen by introducing an R44Q mutation in the coding region of the mouse prostasin gene (*Prss8-R44Q*). It is assumed that this form of prostasin cannot be cleaved and activated, but the serine active site is intact.

Interestingly, all embryos of both transgenic lines survived to term with the expected Mendelian genetic distributions. No apparent anatomic changes were noted in the newborn and the adult mice except for defects in the whisker and pelage hair formation. The matriptase zymogen in the *Prss8-R44Q* mice were cleaved into two chains having a ratio of 30kDa/70kDa similar to that in the control mice, suggesting that the matriptase zymogen cleavage and activation were not affected by having only the prostasin zymogen or an active-site mutant prostasin in mice.

The nephrotic syndrome is a kidney disorder, in which the kidney's glomerular filtration barrier is disrupted, resulting in renal sodium retention and abnormal plasma protein leakage through the glomerulus into the urine.

Prostasin regulates the ENaC to maintain Na^+ homeostasis. By introducing the active-site mutant prostasin (*Prss8-S238A*) or the zymogen locked mutant prostasin (*Prss8-R44Q*) into mice and followed by treating with doxorubicine to mimic the nephrotic syndrome, it was found that the proteolytic ENaC activation and sodium retention are independent of the prostasin form, zymogen-locked, or active-site inactivated[27]. Interestingly, in the same model where the mice were fed with diets of different sodium contents, prostasin zymogen activation is required for a proper ENaC activation[28].

In 2022, Ehret and colleagues[29] generated a mouse model with a targeted prostasin gene inactivation in the kidney. The transgenic mice were generated by crossing mice harboring a transgene of *Prss8[lox/lox]*; *Pax8-rTA[tg/0]*; or *TRE-LC1[tg/0]*. The *Pax8* promoter is active in all tubular cells of the kidney but not in other major organs[30,31], and directs the expression of the reverse tetracycline-dependent transactivator (rtTA). When tetracycline or the analog doxycycline is present, rTA produced in the mouse kidney binds to and activates the responsive promoter that drives the expression of the Cre recombinase (LC-1). The prostasin gene is flanked by the *loxP* sites and is excised by the Cre recombinase (LC-1) in the tubules of the kidney, resulting in a kidney-specific inducible prostasin KO in the mice.

Transgenic mice lacking prostasin expression in the kidney do not show an impaired ENaC-mediated Na⁺ homeostasis or an impaired proteolytic ENaC activation. These studies suggest that prostasin is dispensable in the mouse kidney. While ENaC activation in the kidney is not dependent on the presence of prostasin, the compensatory pathways that regulate the Na⁺ and K⁺ balance may be at play.

15.8 Inhibitors

Inhibitors of serine proteases are grouped into the Kunitz, Kazal, serpin, and mucus families[32]. Studies have shown that prostasin can be inhibited by the Kunitz type inhibitors and the serpins.

Kunitz type inhibitors — natural and reversible

The Kunitz type inhibitor is a competitive serine protease inhibitor containing one or two Kunitz domains, recognized by Kunitz and Northrop[33] in 1936. The Kunitz domain is usually 50–60 amino acid residues in length and interacts with the active site of serine proteases. The prototypical Kunitz protease inhibitor is the bovine pancreatic trypsin inhibitor (BPTI, aka aprotinin) which inhibits both the trypsin-like and the chymotrypsin-like serine proteases. Aprotinin is a non-human naturally occurring serine protease inhibitor and was discovered in the bovine pancreas in 1936 and extracted from the bovine lung in 1964. The mature aprotinin molecule has only 58 amino acid residues stabilized by three disulfide bonds.

Aprotinin is also a drug, sold with the trade name Trasylol, initially developed by Bayer (Germany). It is used clinically to treat acute pancreatitis or to inhibit serine protease activities to reduce bleeding after cardiac surgery. *In vitro*, aprotinin is used as an inhibitor in cell lysis or tissue homogenization to prevent enzymatic degradation of the cellular protein contents intended for measurements in experiments. When coupled to solid resins, e.g., agarose, the aprotinin-agarose is used in chromatography to isolate or remove serine proteases from crude samples. Prostasin is very sensitive to aprotinin inhibition with the half maximal inhibitory concentration (IC_{50}) at 1.8 nM and can be purified by aprotinin-agarose due to the reversibility of the interaction with aprotinin[34].

Application of aprotinin to various epithelial cells, including the A6 Xenopus kidney cells, the JME/CF 15 human nasal epithelial cells, and the M-1 mouse kidney collecting duct cells, results in a reduction of the Na^+ current via the inhibition of various serine proteases such as prostasin, matriptase, plasmin, etc. Therefore, aprotinin has a broad protease spectrum and a lack of specificity to any single serine protease.

The hepatocyte growth factor activator inhibitors HAI-1 (SPINT1) and HAI-2 (SPINT2) are integral and single-transmembrane proteins, each with two Kunitz domains in the extracellular space[35]. The main function of HAI-1 or HAI-2 is to inhibit the hepatocyte growth factor (HGF) activator, a serine protease of the S1 peptidase family, preventing the conversion of the HGF to its active form. The HGF is a tumor-promoting growth factor.

The HAI-1 protein was first purified from the cell culture media of the MKN45 human stomach carcinoma cell line, while the HAI-2 protein was first purified from human placenta, both as inhibitors of the hepatocyte growth factor activator (HGFA)[36,37]. Both inhibitors also inhibit many other serine proteases such as prostasin and matriptase.

Each molecule of HAI-1 or HAI-2 contains two Kunitz domains, KD1 and KD2. The HAI-1 molecule itself can inhibit or reduce its own inhibitory activity towards the target enzyme HGFA via KD2, leaving KD1 as the only functional unit[38,39]. HAI-2, on the other hand, has both KD1 and KD2 as the functional units, but mutations in KD2 could affect the inhibitory efficiency towards prostasin while not matriptase, suggesting that both KD1 and KD2 are required to inhibit prostasin. Mutations in the HAI-2 KD2 have been suggested to be one of the molecular mechanisms in the syndromic congenital sodium diarrhea (SCSD)[40-42].

The interaction of HAI-1 or HAI-2 with prostasin or matriptase has been well studied *in vitro* and *in vivo*. The consensus is that the HAIs are essential physiological regulators of the prostasin and matriptase activities (Figure 15-2). The preference of the enzyme inhibition by either HAI depends on the cellular location of the enzymes and inhibitors

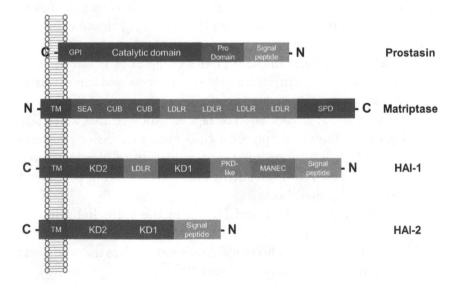

Figure 15-2. Schematic drawing of the membrane anchorage and domains of prostasin, matriptase, HAI-1 and HAI-2. The signal peptide is shown to illustrate orientation, but not present in the mature proteins.

and the types of tissue. The cellular expression and localization of HAIs are spatially regulated. HAI-1 is localized primarily at the cell surface while HAI-2 is mainly seen intracellularly in the granules/vesicles-like structures. For example, HAI-2 is suggested to mainly target prostasin in human intestinal enterocytes intracellularly and near the apical surface, while HAI-1 targets matriptase near the intercellular junctions between enterocytes[40].

It is possible that the complex of HAI-2 with matriptase or prostasin is formed inside the cell and travels to the cell surface. Thereafter, an inhibitor switch may happen, exchanging the bound matriptase or prostasin from HAI-2 to HAI-1. HAI-2 can be shuffled back inside the cell while matriptase or prostasin is localized at the cell surface in a complex with HAI-1. However, the fact that the complexes of the HAIs with either matriptase or prostasin are identified and isolated from the human milk[43] suggests that both inhibitors can form complexes with either enzyme to be released into the bodily fluid, and that the HAIs are physiological regulators of prostasin and matriptase.

Interestingly, when the prostasin protein content increases in cells, the matriptase protein content in those cells is usually down-regulated[44,45], but not vice versa. The HAI-2 binding kinetics and efficiency may favor prostasin over matriptase. HAI-2 may be competed off or depleted from the matriptase-HAI-2 complex by over-expressed prostasin, so the active matriptase may be in excess and can turnover itself and shed from the cell, leaving a reduced quantity in the cell.

Indeed, in 2021, Barndt and colleagues[46] showed that a deletion of HAI-2 in the intestinal epithelial cells causes excessive prostasin proteolysis, which is accompanied by a reduction of matriptase and HAI-1 in these cells. However, such a phenomenon is not prominent in the epidermal epithelial cells.

Down-regulating HAI-1 and HAI-2 in the epithelial cells will up-regulate prostasin and matriptase activities and functions which could lead to diseases and pathological conditions such as the syndromic congenital sodium diarrhea or ichthyosis[41,47].

The HAIs form a complex with either prostasin or matriptase but not both enzymes on the same complex, as suggested by Lai and colleagues[43] in 2016, while an *in vitro* study suggested that HAI-I could form a complex with both prostasin and matriptase at the same time, implying a complex between the two enzymes is structurally possible[48].

Serpin

Serpin is a contracted word of <u>ser</u>ine protease <u>in</u>hibitor. A serpin is an irreversible inhibitor which permanently inactivates a single protease. It is also called a suicide inhibitor because it can only function once. Therefore, the binding of a serpin and its target enzyme is usually at a 1:1 stoichiometry.

Unlike the Kunitz-type inhibitors that reversibly bind to their substrate protease in a lock-and-key Laskowski mechanism, serpins are a family of proteins which use the reactive center loop (RCL) as the substrate-mimicking peptide to antagonize the activity of the protease. The protease cleaves the RCL as they would cleave the enzyme's substrate, but the cleavage triggers a profound conformation change, leading to two ensuing events. The cleaved RCL tucks into the inhibitor and a small fragment of the inhibitor carboxyl-terminus is released from the protease-inhibitor complex. The inhibition is irreversible to the protease. Prostasin (~40 kDa) binds to the serpin protease nexin-1 (PN-1, ~45 kDa) and forms a covalent complex of ~82 kDa, as seen on an SDS-PAGE under reducing conditions, with the release of a small PN-1 fragment[49].

PN-1 was first identified as a component released from normal human foreskin cells. PN-1 forms a covalent complex with the serine protease thrombin or urokinase, regulating the serine protease activity at the cell surface and in the extracellular environment[50]. In 1986, Gioor and colleagues[51] isolated a human cDNA of the glia-derived neurite promoting factor (GdNPF), analysis of the deduced amino acid sequence of the GdNPF cDNA suggested that the GdNPF is the previously identified PN-1, also named as SERPINE2.

Unlike the well-known serpins such as alpha-1 antitrypsin, PN-1 is not made in the liver nor circulating in the blood, rather it is associated with various cells at the cell surface via binding to the glycosaminoglycans (GAGs). It is the fastest thrombin inhibitor among all other serpins with a rate of inhibition at $1 \times 10^6 M^{-1} s^{-1}$ and $\sim 10^9 M^{-1} s^{-1}$ in the presence of the GAGs such as heparin[52]. In mice, PN-1 is predominately expressed in the seminal vesicle, which was the source of the purified PN-1 to show that it binds to prostasin and inhibits the prostasin serine protease activity[49,53].

In 2006, Wakida and colleagues[54] performed experiments to show that small interfering RNA specific to PN-1 was able to reduce the PN-1 expression in the M1 mouse cortical collecting duct cell line. Accordingly, the amiloride-sensitive equivalent current was increased by 60%, presumably by lifting the inhibitory action to the ENaC-activating serine proteases, including prostasin. PN-1 was found to be up-regulated by TGFβ, but down-regulated by aldosterone treatment, adding another layer of control to the ENaC activity.

In 2008, Myerburg and colleagues[55] reported that PN-1 could be a regulator of the matriptase-prostasin cascade in cultured mouse cortical collecting duct cells using the amiloride-sensitive sodium current (I_{Na}) as the readout.

Synthetic inhibitors — Camostat mesilate and nafamostat mesilate

They are synthetic trypsin-like serine protease inhibitors with a broad target spectrum and used for anti-coagulation, anti-inflammation, or anti-viral activities.

From the stem of the word[56] mostat, they belong to proteolytic enzyme inhibitors (INN). The mechanism of action is not clear, but they may do so as a tight-binding substrate occupying the oxyanion hole of the serine protease active site and holding the target enzyme in the acryl-enzyme intermediate form.

They are developed for treating pancreatitis and disseminated intravascular coagulation. The side effects are hyponatremia (low Na^+ in the blood) and hyperkalemia (high K^+ in the blood), possibly due to the inhibition of serine proteases, e.g., prostasin, resulting in a decreased amiloride-sensitive Na^+ conductance, thus less Na^+ reabsorbed.

In 2003, Iwashita and colleagues[57] showed that nafamostat mesilate (NM) reduced the renal sodium reabsorption in rats. Continued infusion of NM into rats resulted in a substantial decrease in the urinary prostasin and urinary sodium excretion.

In 2009, Maekawa and colleagues[58] investigated the camostat mesylate effects in Dahl salt-sensitive rats which develop high blood pressure when fed with a high-salt diet. Oral administration of camostat mesilate reduces the blood pressure in these rats and elevates the urinary Na^+/K^+ ratio. When tested in the M-1 mouse kidney cortical collecting duct cells, camostat mesylate itself does not reduce prostasin expression, rather it inhibits the protease activity of prostasin to reduce the ENaC activity.

In 2009, Coote and colleagues[59] confirmed that camostat inhibited the amiloride-sensitive sodium current in human lung airway epithelial cells.

In 2013, Rowe and colleagues[60] conducted a human study to evaluate the pharmacodynamics, safety, and pharmacokinetics of camostat. Application of camostat through a nasal spray pump to cystic fibrosis (CF) patients was conducted in a randomized, double-blind, placebo-controlled, crossover, ascending single-dose study. It was concluded that camostat can reduce the Na^+ transport in the cystic fibrotic airway via the inhibition of prostasin activity, raising the possibility of targeting prostasin to treat CF. However, the adverse side effects and the poor tolerability may be a concern and require further studies.

Recently, camostat mesylate is explored for its inhibitory activity on TMPRSS2, a key serine protease in potentiating the SARS-CoV-2 infection. The inhibitor could be administered against pneumonia in COVID-19 patients, but the efficacy is questionable in two reported studies[61,62].

References

1. Tully DC, Vidal A, Chatterjee AK, Williams JA, Roberts MJ, Petrassi HM, Spraggon G, Bursulaya B, Pacoma R, Shipway A, Schumacher AM, Danahay H, Harris JL (2008). Discovery of inhibitors of the channel-activating protease prostasin (CAP1/PRSS8) utilizing structure-based design. *Bioorg Med Chem Lett.* 18(22):5895–5899.
2. Shipway A, Danahay H, Williams JA, Tully DC, Backes BJ, Harris JL (2004). Biochemical characterization of prostasin, a channel activating protease. *Biochem Biophys Res Commun.* 324(2):953–963.

3. Edwards PD, Meyer EF Jr, Vijayalakshmi J, Tuthill PA, Andisik DA, Gomes B, Strimpler A (1992). Design, synthesis, and kinetic evaluation of a unique class of elastase inhibitors, the peptidyl .alpha.-ketobenzoxazoles, and the x-ray crystal structure of the covalent complex between porcine pancreatic elastase and Ac-Ala-Pro-Val-2-benzoxazole. *J Am Chem Soc.* 114(5):1854–1863.

4. Maryanoff BE, Costanzo MJ (2008). Inhibitors of proteases and amide hydrolases that employ an α-ketoheterocycle as a key enabling functionality. *Bioorg & Med Chem.* 16(4):1562–1595.

5. Garty H, Palmer LG (1997). Epithelial sodium channels: Function, structure, and regulation. *Physiol Rev.* 77(2):359–396.

6. Chraïbi A, Horisberger JD (2002). Na self inhibition of human epithelial Na channel: temperature dependence and effect of extracellular proteases. *J Gen Physiol.* 120(2):133–145.

7. Bize V, Horisberger JD (2007). Sodium self-inhibition of human epithelial sodium channel: Selectivity and affinity of the extracellular sodium sensing site. *Am J Physiol Renal Physiol.* 293(4):F1137–F1146.

8. Bhalla V, Hallows KR (2008). Mechanisms of ENaC regulation and clinical implications. *J Am Soc Nephrol.* 19(10):1845–1854.

9. Chen M, Chen LM, Lin CY, Chai KX (2008). The epidermal growth factor receptor (EGFR) is proteolytically modified by the Matriptase-Prostasin serine protease cascade in cultured epithelial cells. *Biochim Biophys Acta.* 1783(5):896–903.

10. Chen M, Chen LM, Lin CY, Chai KX (2010). Hepsin activates prostasin and cleaves the extracellular domain of the epidermal growth factor receptor. *Mol Cell Biochem.* 337(1–2):259–266.

11. Chen LM, Chai KX (2017). Proteolytic cleavages in the extracellular domain of receptor tyrosine kinases by membrane-associated serine proteases. *Oncotarget.* 8(34):56490–56505.

12. Chen M, Fu YY, Lin CY, Chen LM, Chai KX (2007). Prostasin induces protease-dependent and independent molecular changes in the human prostate carcinoma cell line PC-3. *Biochim Biophys Acta.* 1773(7):113–140.

13. Heuberger DM, Schuepbach RA (2019). Protease-activated receptors (PARs): Mechanisms of action and potential therapeutic modulators in PAR-driven inflammatory diseases. *Thromb J.* 17:4. Erratum in: *Thromb J.* 2019 Nov 6;17:22.

14. Chen LM, Hatfield ML, Fu YY, Chai KX (2009). Prostasin regulates iNOS and cyclin D1 expression by modulating protease-activated receptor-2 signaling in prostate epithelial cells. *Prostate.* 69(16):1790–1801.

15. Camerer E, Barker A, Duong DN, Ganesan R, Kataoka H, Cornelissen I, Darragh MR, Hussain A, Zheng YW, Srinivasan Y, Brown C, Xu SM, Regard JB, Lin CY, Craik CS, Kirchhofer D, Coughlin SR (2010). Local protease signaling contributes to neural tube closure in the mouse embryo. *Dev Cell.* 18(1):25–38.

16. Friis S, Tadeo D, Le-Gall SM, Jürgensen HJ, Sales KU, Camerer E, Bugge TH (2017). Matriptase zymogen supports epithelial development, homeostasis and regeneration. *BMC Biol.* 15(1):46.

17. Frateschi S, Camerer E, Crisante G, Rieser S, Membrez M, Charles RP, Beermann F, Stehle JC, Breiden B, Sandhoff K, Rotman S, Haftek M, Wilson A, Ryser S, Steinhoff M, Coughlin SR, Hummler E (2011). PAR2 absence completely rescues inflammation and ichthyosis caused by altered CAP1/Prss8 expression in mouse skin. *Nat Commun.* 2:161.

18. Chen LM, Wang C, Chen M, Marcello MR, Chao J, Chao L, Chai KX (2006). Prostasin attenuates inducible nitric oxide synthase expression in lipopolysaccharide-induced urinary bladder inflammation. *Am J Physiol Renal Physiol.* 291(3):F567–F577.

19. Uchimura K, Hayata M, Mizumoto T, Miyasato Y, Kakizoe Y, Morinaga J, Onoue T, Yamazoe R, Ueda M, Adachi M, Miyoshi T, Shiraishi N, Ogawa W, Fukuda K, Kondo T, Matsumura T, Araki E, Tomita K, Kitamura K (2014). The serine protease prostasin regulates hepatic insulin sensitivity by modulating TLR4 signalling. *Nat Commun.* 5:3428.

20. Sugitani Y, Nishida A, Inatomi O, Ohno M, Imai T, Kawahara M, Kitamura K, Andoh A (2020). Sodium absorption stimulator prostasin (PRSS8) has an anti-inflammatory effect via downregulation of TLR4 signaling in inflammatory bowel disease. *J Gastroenterol.* 55(4): 408–417.

21. Murray AS, Hyland TE, Sala-Hamrick KE, Mackinder JR, Martin CE, Tanabe LM, Varela FA, List K (2020). The cell-surface anchored serine protease TMPRSS13 promotes breast cancer progression and resistance to chemotherapy. *Oncogene.* 39(41):6421–6436.

22. Netzel-Arnett S, Currie BM, Szabo R, Lin CY, Chen LM, Chai KX, Antalis TM, Bugge TH, List K (2006). Evidence for a matriptase-prostasin proteolytic cascade regulating terminal epidermal differentiation. *J Biol Chem.* 281(44):32941–32945.

23. Hummler E, Dousse A, Rieder A, Stehle JC, Rubera I, Osterheld MC, Beermann F, Frateschi S, Charles RP (2013). The channel-activating protease CAP1/Prss8 is required for placental labyrinth maturation. *PLoS One.* 8(2):e55796.

24. List K, Haudenschild CC, Szabo R, Chen W, Wahl SM, Swaim W, Engelholm LH, Behrendt N, Bugge TH (2002). Matriptase/MT-SP1 is required for postnatal survival, epidermal barrier function, hair follicle development, and thymic homeostasis. *Oncogene.* 21(23):3765–3779.

25. Peters DE, Szabo R, Friis S, Shylo NA, Uzzun Sales K, Holmbeck K, Bugge TH (2014). The membrane-anchored serine protease prostasin (CAP1/ PRSS8) supports epidermal development and postnatal homeostasis independent of its enzymatic activity. *J Biol Chem.* 289(21):14740–14749.

26. Friis S, Madsen DH, Bugge TH (2016). Distinct developmental functions of prostasin (CAP1/PRSS8) zymogen and activated prostasin. *J Biol Chem.* 291(6):2577–2582.

27. Essigke D, Bohnert BN, Janessa A, Wörn M, Omage K, Kalbacher H, Birkenfeld AL, Bugge TH, Szabo R, Artunc F (2022). Sodium retention in nephrotic syndrome is independent of the activation of the membrane-anchored serine protease prostasin (CAP1/PRSS8) and its enzymatic activity. *Pflugers Arch.* 474(6):613–624.

28. Essigke D, Ilyaskin AV, Wörn M, Bohnert BN, Xiao M, Daniel C, Amann K, Birkenfeld AL, Szabo R, Bugge TH, Korbmacher C, Artunc F (2021). Zymogen-locked mutant prostasin (Prss8) leads to incomplete proteolytic activation of the epithelial sodium channel (ENaC) and severely compromises triamterene tolerance in mice. *Acta Physiol (Oxf).* 232(1):e13640.

29. Ehret E, Jäger Y, Sergi C, Mérillat AM, Peyrollaz T, Anand D, Wang Q, Ino F, Maillard M, Kellenberger S, Gautschi I, Szabo R, Bugge TH, Vogel LK, Hummler E, Frateschi S (2022). Kidney-specific CAP1/Prss8-deficient mice maintain ENaC-mediated sodium balance through an aldosterone independent pathway. *Int J Mol Sci.* 23(12):6745.

30. Plachov D, Chowdhury K, Walther C, Simon D, Guenet JL, Gruss P (1990). Pax8, a murine paired box gene expressed in the developing excretory system and thyroid gland. *Development.* 110(2):643–651.

31. Traykova-Brauch M, Schönig K, Greiner O, Miloud T, Jauch A, Bode M, Felsher DW, Glick AB, Kwiatkowski DJ, Bujard H, Horst J, von Knebel Doeberitz M, Niggli FK, Kriz W, Gröne HJ, Koesters R (2008). An efficient and versatile system for acute and chronic modulation of renal tubular function in transgenic mice. *Nat Med.* 14(9):979–984.

32. Roberts RM, Mathialagan N, Duffy JY, Smith GW (1995). Regulation and regulatory role of proteinase inhibitors. *Crit Rev Eukaryot Gene Expr.* 5(3-4):385–436.

33. Kunitz M, Northrop JH (1936). Isolation from beef pancreas of crystalline trypsinogen, trypsin, a trypsin inhibitor, and an inhibitor-trypsin compound. *J Gen Physiol.* 19(6):991–1007.

34. Yu JX, Chao L, Chao J (1994). Prostasin is a novel human serine proteinase from seminal fluid. Purification, tissue distribution, and localization in prostate gland. *J Biol Chem.* 269(29):18843–18848.

35. Kataoka H, Kawaguchi M, Fukushima T, Shimomura T (2018). Hepatocyte growth factor activator inhibitors (HAI-1 and HAI-2): Emerging key players in epithelial integrity and cancer. *Pathol Int.* 68(3):145–158.

36. Shimomura T, Denda K, Kitamura A, Kawaguchi T, Kito M, Kondo J, Kagaya S, Qin L, Takata H, Miyazawa K, Kitamura N (1997). Hepatocyte growth factor activator inhibitor, a novel Kunitz-type serine protease inhibitor. *J Biol Chem.* 272(10):6370–6376.

37. Marlor CW, Delaria KA, Davis G, Muller DK, Greve JM, Tamburini PP (1997). Identification and cloning of human placental bikunin, a novel serine protease inhibitor containing two Kunitz domains. *J Biol Chem.* 272(18):12202–12208.

38. Denda K, Shimomura T, Kawaguchi T, Miyazawa K, Kitamura N (2002). Functional characterization of Kunitz domains in hepatocyte growth factor activator inhibitor type 1. *J Biol Chem.* 277(16):14053–14059.

39. Liu M, Yuan C, Jensen JK, Zhao B, Jiang Y, Jiang L, Huang M (2017). The crystal structure of a multidomain protease inhibitor (HAI-1) reveals the mechanism of its auto-inhibition. *J Biol Chem.* 292(20):8412–8423. Erratum in: *J Biol Chem.* 2017 Jun 23;292(25):10744.

40. Shiao F, Liu LO, Huang N, Lai YJ, Barndt RJ, Tseng CC, Wang JK, Jia B, Johnson MD, Lin CY (2017). Selective inhibition of prostasin in human enterocytes by the integral membrane kunitz-type serine protease inhibitor HAI-2. *PLoS One.* 12(1):e0170944.

41. Holt-Danborg L, Vodopiutz J, Nonboe AW, De Laffolie J, Skovbjerg S, Wolters VM, Müller T, Hetzer B, Querfurt A, Zimmer KP, Jensen JK, Entenmann A, Heinz-Erian P, Vogel LK, Janecke AR (2019). SPINT2 (HAI-2) missense variants identified in congenital sodium diarrhea/tufting enteropathy affect the ability of HAI-2 to inhibit prostasin but not matriptase. *Hum Mol Genet.* 28(5):828–841.

42. Skovbjerg S, Holt-Danborg L, Nonboe AW, Hong Z, Frost ÁK, Schar CR, Thomas CC, Vitved L, Jensen JK, Vogel LK (2020). Inhibition of an active zymogen protease: The zymogen form of matriptase is regulated by HAI-1 and HAI-2. *Biochem J.* 477(9):1779–1794.

43. Lai CH, Lai YJ, Chou FP, Chang HH, Tseng CC, Johnson MD, Wang JK, Lin CY (2016). Matriptase complexes and prostasin complexes with HAI-1 and HAI-2 in human milk: Significant proteolysis in lactation. *PLoS One.* 11(4):e0152904.

44. Buzza MS, Martin EW, Driesbaugh KH, Désilets A, Leduc R, Antalis TM (2013). Prostasin is required for matriptase activation in intestinal epithelial cells to regulate closure of the paracellular pathway. *J Biol Chem.* 288(15):10328–10337.

45. Chai AC, Robinson AL, Chai KX, Chen LM (2015). Ibuprofen regulates the expression and function of membrane-associated serine proteases prostasin and matriptase. *BMC Cancer.* 15:1025.

46. Barndt RB, Lee MJ, Huang N, Lu DD, Lee SC, Du PW, Chang CC, Tsai PB, Huang YK, Chang HM, Wang JK, Lai CH, Johnson MD, Lin CY (2021). Targeted HAI-2 deletion causes excessive proteolysis with prolonged active prostasin and depletion of HAI-1 monomer in intestinal but not epidermal epithelial cells. *Hum Mol Genet.* 30(19):1833–1850.

47. Nagaike K, Kawaguchi M, Takeda N, Fukushima T, Sawaguchi A, Kohama K, Setoyama M, Kataoka H (2008). Defect of hepatocyte growth factor activator inhibitor type 1/serine protease inhibitor, Kunitz type 1 (Hai-1/Spint1) leads to ichthyosis-like condition and abnormal hair development in mice. *Am J Pathol.* 173(5):1464–1475.

48. Friis S, Uzzun Sales K, Godiksen S, Peters DE, Lin CY, Vogel LK, Bugge TH (2013). A matriptase-prostasin reciprocal zymogen activation complex with unique features: Prostasin as a non-enzymatic co-factor for matriptase activation. *J Biol Chem.* 288(26):19028–19039.

49. Chen LM, Zhang X, Chai KX (2004). Regulation of prostasin expression and function in the prostate. *Prostate.* 59(1):1–12.

50. Baker JB, Low DA, Simmer RL, Cunningham DD (1980). Protease-nexin: a cellular component that links thrombin and plasminogen activator and mediates their binding to cells. *Cell.* 21(1):37–45.

51. Gloor S, Odink K, Guenther J, Nick H, Denis Monard D (1986). A glia-derived neurite promoting factor with protease inhibitory activity belongs to the protease nexins. *Cell.* 47(5):687–693.

52. Li W, Huntington JA (2012). Crystal structures of protease nexin-1 in complex with heparin and thrombin suggest a 2-step recognition mechanism. *Blood.* 120(2):459–467.

53. Vassalli JD, Huarte J, Bosco D, Sappino AP, Sappino N, Velardi A, Wohlwend A, Ernø H, Monard D, Belin D (1993). Protease-nexin I as an

androgen-dependent secretory product of the murine seminal vesicle. *EMBO J.* 12(5):1871–1878.

54. Wakida N, Kitamura K, Tuyen DG, Maekawa A, Miyoshi T, Adachi M, Shiraishi N, Ko T, Ha V, Nonoguchi H, Tomita K (2006). Inhibition of prostasin-induced ENaC activities by PN-1 and regulation of PN-1 expression by TGF-beta1 and aldosterone. *Kidney Int.* 70(8):1432–1438.

55. Myerburg MM, McKenna EE, Luke CJ, Frizzell RA, Kleyman TR, Pilewski JM (2008). Prostasin expression is regulated by airway surface liquid volume and is increased in cystic fibrosis. *Am J Physiol Lung Cell Mol Physiol.* 294(5):L932–L941.

56. World Health Organization (2018). The use of stems in the selection of International Nonproprietary Names (INN) for pharmaceutical substances.

57. Iwashita K, Kitamura K, Narikiyo T, Adachi M, Shiraishi N, Miyoshi T, Nagano J, Tuyen DG, Nonoguchi H, Tomita K (2003). Inhibition of prostasin secretion by serine protease inhibitors in the kidney. *J Am Soc Nephrol.* 14(1):11–16.

58. Maekawa A, Kakizoe Y, Miyoshi T, Wakida N, Ko T, Shiraishi N, Adachi M, Tomita K, Kitamura K (2009). Camostat mesilate inhibits prostasin activity and reduces blood pressure and renal injury in salt-sensitive hypertension. *J Hypertens.* 27(1):181189.

59. Coote K, Atherton-Watson HC, Sugar R, Young A, MacKenzie-Beevor A, Gosling M, Bhalay G, Bloomfield G, Dunstan A, Bridges RJ, Sabater JR, Abraham WM, Tully D, Pacoma R, Schumacher A, Harris J, Danahay H (2009). Camostat attenuates airway epithelial sodium channel function in vivo through the inhibition of a channel-activating protease. *J Pharmacol Exp Ther.* 329(2):764–774.

60. Rowe SM, Reeves G, Hathorne H, Solomon GM, Abbi S, Renard D, Lock R, Zhou P, Danahay H, Clancy JP, Waltz DA (2013). Reduced sodium transport with nasal administration of the prostasin inhibitor camostat in subjects with cystic fibrosis. *Chest.* 144(1):200–207.

61. Gunst JD, Staerke NB, Pahus MH, Kristensen LH, Bodilsen J, Lohse N, Dalgaard LS, Brønnum D, Fröbert O, Hønge B, Johansen IS, Monrad I, Erikstrup C, Rosendal R, Vilstrup E, Mariager T, Bove DG, Offersen R, Shakar S, Cajander S, Jørgensen NP, Sritharan SS, Breining P, Jespersen S, Mortensen KL, Jensen ML, Kolte L, Frattari GS, Larsen CS, Storgaard M, Nielsen LP, Tolstrup M, Sædder EA, Østergaard LJ, Ngo

HTT, Jensen MH, Højen JF, Kjolby M, Søgaard OS (2021). Efficacy of the TMPRSS2 inhibitor camostat mesilate in patients hospitalized with Covid-19-a double-blind randomized controlled trial. *EClinicalMedicine*. 35:100849.

62. Tobback E, Degroote S, Buysse S, Delesie L, Van Dooren L, Vanherrewege S, Barbezange C, Hutse V, Romano M, Thomas I, Padalko E, Callens S, De Scheerder MA (2022). Efficacy and safety of camostat mesylate in early COVID-19 disease in an ambulatory setting: A randomized placebo-controlled phase II trial. *Int J Infect Dis*. 122:628–635.

Chapter 16

Prostasin as a Biomarker, a Drug Target, and in Therapeutic Development

A biomarker is defined as "a measurable substance in an organism whose presence is indicative of some phenomenon such as disease, infection, or environmental exposure" (Oxford Languages). Biomarkers are divided into seven categories including susceptibility/risk biomarker, diagnostic biomarker, monitoring biomarker, prognostic biomarker, predictive biomarker, response biomarker, and safety biomarker [BEST (Biomarkers, EndpointS, and other Tools) Resource]. The easily accessible sample sources for biomarker measurements can be the blood, urine, saliva, and other bodily fluids, or soft tissues.

As we have discussed in the preceding chapters, prostasin as a membrane-anchored extracellular serine protease has important and vital roles in the tissues and organs of the body from the embryonic development to the mature adult, and onto the reproduction cycle. Its expression is regulated by numerous environmental factors such as growth factors and cytokines, as well as cellular and molecular pathways such as the SREBPs (sterol-regulatory element-binding proteins). The prostasin gene is also susceptible to epigenetic regulation involving promoter DNA methylation and histone modifications. Biochemically, the prostasin protein can be shed off by the actions of phospholipases or exported as a membrane component in the exosomes. These qualities would seem to suggest that prostasin could serve as a molecular marker, a drug target, or a therapeutic agent. However, currently prostasin is not used as a biomarker in any of the above categories, rather prostasin has been and is still being evaluated, either alone or in combination with other proteins, in various diseases or conditions for its potential as a biomarker.

16.1 The urinary prostasin

The human urine was determined to contain the prostasin protein at about 0.2 µg/ml[1] and this bodily fluid is easily collected for measurements. However, the urinary prostasin could come from the epithelial cells along the entire urinary tract including the kidney, ureter, bladder, and urethra, or possibly be adulterated by mixing with semen in males. The prostasin present in the urine could be exported actively by the epithelium along the urinary tract, or the result of tissue damage. In either case, an evaluation of the urinary prostasin level may provide the information on the health of the urinary tract and even the whole body.

With the understanding that prostasin activates the epithelial sodium channel (ENaC) in the kidney, physiologically, with the influence of the renin-angiotensin-aldosterone system, the prostasin content and its changes in human urine have been investigated in various human populations and by various means.

In 2002, Narikiyo and colleagues[2] examined prostasin secretion in the urine by means of electrophoresis and immunoblotting and reported a higher urinary prostasin level in primary aldosteronism subjects when compared to control subjects. This high level of the urinary prostasin could be reduced back to normal levels after adrenalectomy, removal of the adrenal glands that produce aldosterone. The authors suggested that aldosterone may regulate prostasin expression and secretion.

In 2005, with the same method, Olivieri and colleagues[3] reported that the urinary prostasin decreased after spironolactone treatment in normotensives with a low sodium diet but not a high sodium diet. The urinary prostasin decreased in the normotensive after saline infusion, but increased in primary aldosteronism after volume expansion. The authors suggested that two portions of urinary prostasin exist, the basal/constitutively secreted and the aldosterone-responsive secreted portions. The latter is potentially suitable as a surrogate marker for activation of the kidney ENaC because this portion is modulated by sodium intake.

In 2009, Koda and colleagues[4] developed a radioimmunoassay (RIA) specific to the human prostasin and analysed the level of urinary prostasin, which was strongly correlated with the level of aldosterone in the urine, or in the plasma. However, the excretion of prostasin is inversely correlated with the urinary Na^+/K^+ ratio.

In the same year, Zhu and colleagues[5] determined the urinary prostasin level by means of enzyme-linked immunosorbent assay (ELISA) in subjects who participated in a behavioural stress-induced pressure natriuresis (SIPN) model and reported that the baseline level of the urinary prostasin is at 38.4 ng/ml, while it decreased during the stress period to 17.2 ng/ml, and further declined to 12.1 ng/ml in the recovery period. The excretion of the urinary prostasin was inversely correlated with the secretion of the urinary sodium during the behavioural stress in normotensive adolescents.

In 2013, Olivieri and colleagues[6] measured urinary prostasin levels with an ELISA in normotensive individuals and found that the prostasin content in the urine ranged from 0.5–18.9 nM or 20–756 ng/ml, a rather broad range. The level of prostasin correlated with the aldosterone to renin ratio (ARR), as well as the level of the urinary Na^+. The authors suggested that prostasin is modulated by the urinary Na^+ and appears to be correlated with the ARR rather than with the individual factor, either aldosterone or renin alone in the plasma.

In the same year, Guo and colleagues[7] evaluated the urinary prostasin by ELISA and showed an increased prostasin excretion, coinciding with an aldosterone increase in the plasma, in a human population with adiposity.

In 2015, Andersen and colleagues[8] observed an increased ratio of the urinary prostasin/creatinine in type 1 diabetic individuals with nephropathy (DN) along with a high level of the urinary albumin, while the exosomal prostasin level showed no difference between patients and control subjects. When compared to the controls, the DN patient urine increased the amiloride-sensitive inward Na^+ current of a single M1 mouse collecting duct cell in patch-clamp experiments.

In 2016, Frederiksen-Møller and colleagues[9] reported an increased prostasin level in the urine from pregnant women with preeclampsia, while Zheng and colleagues[10] reported an increased urinary prostasin level in chronic heart failure (CHF) patients. Similarly, the urine from the CHF patients increased the inward Na⁺ current in the M1 cells as well.

In 2017, Pizzolo and colleagues[11] measured the urinary prostasin level by ELISA in patients with primary aldosteronism and essential hypertension and found that the urinary prostasin level is higher in primary aldosteronism than that in essential hypertension patients. However, further data analysis using a receiver operating characteristic (ROC) curve indicated a poor sensitivity (true positive rate) if prostasin were used as a diagnostic marker for primary aldosteronism, even though specific.

In 2017, Oxlund and colleagues[12] analyzed the prostasin content in the urine of patients having type 2 diabetes with treatment-resistant hypertension and reported that the ratio of prostasin/creatinine was similar in the urine with or without the spironolactone treatment. By means of western blotting, prostasin was detected in samples with albuminuria but barely in samples without albuminuria. The urinary prostasin level decreased following the spironolactone treatment when compared to the placebo subjects, but this result may be due to the overall improved glomerular filtration barrier function and reduced proteinuria. Activation of the aldosterone pathway did not have a direct effect on the abundance of prostasin in the urine and kidney tissues, as discussed by the authors.

In 2018, Hinrichs and colleagues[13] used western blotting for urinary prostasin determination in kidney transplant recipients (KTR) with or without albuminuria. The amount of the urinary prostasin was usually found at a higher level and is significantly correlated with albuminuria in the KTRs. The urine from the KTRs with albuminuria could activate the amiloride- and aprotinin-sensitive inward Na⁺ current of the M1 mouse kidney collecting duct cells. In line with this, the ENaC γ-subunit in the urinary exosomes was in the cleaved form, and more in quantity in the KTRs with albuminuria when compared to those without albuminuria, indicating a potential increase of proteolytic activation of the ENaC in the kidney of transplant recipients with albuminuria.

Despite the easy access and the efforts made by the research investigations cited above, the urinary prostasin content does not appear to

Table 16-1. Quantification of the prostasin level in human urine. In the right column, the numbers represent the approximate mean values or ranges in the normal/control groups in each study, except that "Type 2" in the parenthesis represents type 2 diabetes with treatment-resistance hypertension before the spironolactone treatment. The top four data groups are expressed as nanogram per milliliter. The bottom three data groups are normalised against the urinary creatinine and expressed as nanogram per milligram. In the middle column, the numbers in the parentheses are the Reference numbers listed at the end of this chapter. The prostasin level in human urine varies with a broad range depending on the detection methods listed in the left column.

Method	Author, Year	Urine (ng/ml)
ELISA, Homemade	Zhu, 2009 (5)	38.4
ELISA, CUSABIO®	Anderson, 2015 (8)	10–50
RIA, Homemade	Yu, 1994 (1)	200
ELISA, Homemade	Olivieri, 2013 (6)	20–756
		Urine (ng/mg)
ELISA, Homemade	Guo, 2013 (7)	20.7
ELISA, CUSABIO®	Oxlund, 2017 (12)	1.0–22.9(Type 2)
ELISA, CUSABIO®	Andersen, 2015 (8)	1.5–30
ELISA, CUSABIO®	Frederiksen-Møller, 2016 (9)	8,200–31,201

be of significance as a biomarker for a condition or disease state, mainly due to the broad range of prostasin levels in the tested populations (Table 16-1).

16.2 The blood prostasin

The blood does not usually have the prostasin protein. If there is, its origin may be the epithelial cells in other organs, as prostasin could be leaked into the blood stream as a soluble protein or in the membrane-bound form by the stressed or injured epithelial tissues. In recent years, prostasin has been selected and incorporated into biomarker panels for association analysis in the disease states. A comparison can be made with the blood biomarker of prostate cancer in the serine protease the prostate-specific antigen (PSA), which is produced by the normal prostate epithelial cells and secreted into the seminal plasma. A disruption of the proper tissue architecture in the prostate as it is in the case of prostate cancer would result in the leakage of this protein to the wrong side of the prostate epithelium and into the blood. The more advanced the cancer, the more extent the tissue architecture disruption and there would be more PSA in the blood.

In 2015, Andersen and colleagues[8] observed an increased plasma prostasin level in type 1 diabetic individuals with nephropathy (DN) when compared to the control subjects. The prostasin level ranged from 6–12 µg/ml, as measured in an ELISA (CUSABIO®).

In 2016, Frederiksen-Møller and colleagues[9] measured prostasin levels in human plasma and did not find significant differences in pregnant women with or without preeclampsia. The plasma prostasin level ranged from about 6–19 µg/ml, as measured in an ELISA (CUSABIO®).

In 2017, Oxlund and colleagues[12] reported that the plasma prostasin level is not correlated with the serum aldosterone concentration in type 2 diabetes patients with treatment-resistant hypertension after spironolactone treatment when compared to that in the placebo group, however, the urinary prostasin did correlated with the serum aldosterone in all subjects before the treatment. The plasma prostasin was measured using the ELISA from CUSABIO® and ranged from 2.8–26.0 µg/ml.

In 2018, Raghu and colleagues[14] suggested a possible association of prostasin with idiopathic pulmonary fibrosis (IPF) by analyzing patients' circulating biomarkers using the Human Discovery Multi-Analyte Profile (MAP) 250+ panel (Myriad RBM, Inc., Austin, TX). IPF is a progressive fibrotic interstitial lung disease that leads to respiratory failure and ultimately death. The etiology of the disease is currently unknown.

In 2019, Lal and colleagues[15] carried out a proteomic analysis using a targeted ELISA for 254 serum proteins (Myriad RBM) and found that prostasin was over-expressed in individuals with the obstructive sleep apnea syndrome (OSAS) with cognitive impairment (CI) when compared to those without CI.

In the same year, Stattin and colleagues[16] reported that the plasma prostasin, along with 74 other plasma marker proteins, is inversely associated with physical activity in two population-based cohorts. The

Olink Proseek Multiplex Cardiovascular II and III panels were used for the plasma protein marker measurements. The plasma prostasin quantity was expressed as log2-normalized protein expression (NPX) values.

In 2021, Pietzner and colleagues[17] analyzed 4,775 protein targets in the plasma from 10,708 European-descent individuals in a genome-proteome-wide association study to create a proteo-genomic human health map with protein-quantitative trait loci (pQTLs). The quantitative variants were tested against the genomic variants at protein-encoding loci (cis-pQTLs). Prostasin (*PRSS8*) was identified to be strongly associated with Alzheimer's disease (AD). In fact, the authors assigned *PRSS8* as a candidate causal gene for Alzheimer's diseases at the *KAT8* locus which was previously identified as one of the 29 AD risk loci by a genome-wide meta-analysis (GWAS). Alzheimer's disease is the most frequent neurodegenerative disease and is highly heritable but no actual causal genes for the disease have been identified.

Almost half of all heart failure cases in the United States are diagnosed as heart failure with preserved ejection fraction (HFpEF), also referred to as diastolic heart failure[18]. In the aldosterone receptor blockade in diastolic heart failure (Aldo-DHF) trial, a multicenter study[19,20], spironolactone was indicated as a potentially effective medication for improving the left ventricular diastolic function in the HFpEF patients. Spironolactone is a potassium-sparing diuretic drug used to treat heart failure, high blood pressure (hypertension), and low blood potassium (hypokalemia). Spironolactone prevents water build up in the body by blocking the mineralocorticoid receptor, the target of mineralocorticoids such as aldosterone.

In 2021, Schnelle and colleagues[21] further analyzed the same cohort (Aldo-DHF) by means of the Olink technology (Olink, Uppsala, Sweden). Ninety-two biomarkers in a pre-selected cardiovascular panel II (CVD II) were measured simultaneously using 1 µl of patient plasma. The log2-normalized protein expression (NPX) values indicated that the prostasin level in the baseline plasma of the HFpEF patients has a predictive value on the treatment effect of a 12-month spironolactone course based on the criteria of spironolactone-mediated effects on the relative peak VO_2, the highest oxygen achieved during the cardiopulmonary exercise testing. Interestingly, spironolactone treatment could increase the plasma prostasin level in type 2 diabetic patients with treatment-resistant hypertension[12].

In a study carried out by Cauwenberghs and colleagues[22] in 2021, prostasin was identified as one of the top 13 pathologically relevant proteins associated with echocardiographic abnormalities in the early stage of heart failure analyzed by the same CVD II panel. Also in 2021, Verdonschot and colleagues[23] applied the Olink Proseek® Multiplex cardiovascular and inflammation panels with 276 protein biomarkers to compare the proteomic profiles of patients at risk for developing heart failure in the "Heart omics in AGEing" (HOMAGE) trial[24]. It was shown that the baseline prostasin level is higher in the diabetic patients when compared to the non-diabetics, and the prostasin level was not affected by the spironolactone treatment (ClinicalTrials.gov Identifier: NCT02556450). In 2022, Chandramouli and colleagues[25] applied the Olink Proseek® Multiplex cardiovascular II and III, and the inflammation 96×96 kits on patient blood samples and found that prostasin was correlated with heart failure and preserved ejection fraction (HFpEF) with coronary microvascular dysfunction (CMD) among women but not men.

In 2021, Sekine and colleagues[26] reported that the human serum prostasin level is at about 300 pg/ml and is negatively associated with the presence of type 2 diabetes, while Uchimura and colleagues[27] in 2014 reported serum prostasin levels ranging from 0.9–3.4 ng/ml.

In 2022, Bao and colleagues[28] analyzed plasma samples from 6,103 subjects collected over three years in Malmö, Sweden. Among them, 4,658 subjects had complete data on prostasin and covariates, but 361 subjects with prevalent diabetes were excluded. Therefore, 4,297 subjects, 38.5% men, were selected for further analysis. It is worth noting that among this cohort of 4,297 participants, 232 have a history of cancer and 93 have cardiovascular diseases. The plasma prostasin level was measured using the Proseek® Multiplex Oncology I v2 96×96 Panel by means of the Olink technology (Olink Proteomics, Sweden). They reported that the plasma prostasin level may be used as a risk predictor for developing diabetes and for death from cancer especially for those cancer patients with high blood glucose. However, the prostasin level is presented as the NPX, therefore it cannot be used for comparison with other measurements for absolute concentrations. In addition, no Bonferroni correction was performed in this study as the authors discussed. It would be interesting to learn if other proteins in the same testing Panels showed changes along with prostasin.

Finding prostasin in the blood in various conditions could help identify if there were any compromised epithelium and the surrounding architecture in the body, however, the specificity of prostasin as a biomarker in the blood for evaluating a disease status requires further comprehensive investigations. Most important, as the reported blood prostasin levels vary over an incredibly wide range from the different studies by different methods on different populations, the authenticity of the prostasin being measured is desperately in need of validation (Table 16-2). A very high reported level of prostasin presence in the blood is not reconciling with the current landscape of prostasin expression in either normal physiology or pathophysiology. A very low reported level of the blood prostasin will present a big challenge to the specificity of its potential use as a marker as the test accuracy is probably shot.

Table 16-2. Quantification of the prostasin level in human blood. In the right column, the numbers represent the approximate mean values or ranges in the normal/control groups in each study, except that "Type 2" in the parenthesis represents type 2 diabetes with treatment-resistance hypertension before the spironolactone treatment. The prostasin level in human plasma or serum varies with a broad range depending on the detection methods listed in the left column. In the middle column, the numbers in the parentheses are the reference numbers listed at the end of this chapter.

Method	Author, Year	Plasma/Serum (ng/ml)
ELISA, BOSTER Biological Technology Co.	Sekine, 2021 (26)	0.3
RIA, Homemade	Uchimura, 2014 (27)	0.9–3.4
ELISA, MyriadRBM/ xMAP® Technology	Raghu, 2018 (14)	50–600
RIA, Homemade	Bastani, 2017 (56)	7,210
ELISA, CUSABIO®	Andersen, 2015 (8)	6,000–12,000
ELISA, CUSABIO®	Frederiksen-Møller, 2016 (9)	6,000–19,000
ELISA, CUSABIO®	Oxlund, 2017 (12)	2,800–26,000 (Type 2)

16.3 The exosomal prostasin

The exosomes are nanoparticles of 30–150 nm in size, released from cells. The exosomes carry the plasma membrane protein signatures of the cell origin due to the fusion of the multicellular bodies with the cell plasma membrane in the process of forming these extracellular vesicles[29].

In 2012, van der Lubbe and colleagues[30] explored the possibility of using the urinary exosomes for prostasin evaluation in patients with primary aldosteronism and essential hypertension, and reported that the exosomal prostasin was slightly increased in patients with primary aldosteronism, but not statistically significant.

In 2013, Olivieri and colleagues[6] also measured prostasin in the urinary exosomes and indicated that the exosomal prostasin displayed similar patterns as seen with the urinary prostasin.

In 2015, Castagna and colleagues[31] reported that the level of urinary exosomal prostasin changes following a circadian pattern with a low level in the morning and higher levels in the afternoon and evening. Interestingly, that is in an inverse relationship with the circadian pattern of the blood aldosterone level, in which the peak level is in the morning[32].

In 2016, Qi and colleagues[33] examined the urinary exosomes in hypertensive patients under a high-sodium or a low-sodium diet which activates the endogenous renin-angiotensin-aldosterone system. The liquid chromatography-tandem mass spectrometry-based multidimensional protein identification technology was used to analyze the exosome proteins in the urine. A total number of 2,775 unique proteins were identified. Among them, 316 proteins had significant quantity changes during a low salt diet, prostasin was not one of them.

In 2019, Zachar and colleagues[34] reported that the prostasin excreted in the exosome form in the human urine was increased after five days of a low sodium diet, analyzed by western blotting.

In 2021, Krishnamachary and colleagues[35] reported that prostasin was one of the most up-regulated proteins in the plasma exosomes in patients with severe coronavirus disease-2019 (COVID-19). COVID-19

It is very important to point out however, that the commonly accepted p-value for false positives at 0.05 in a clinical case-control study needs to factor in the chance of false positives at all of the SNP sites in a genetic association study. In statistics, the practice is called the Bonferroni correction when several dependent or independent tests are performed simultaneously. The Bonferroni correction sets the p-value for the entire set of "n" comparisons at "p/n". So, the threshold p-value for GWAS is made much more stringent at 0.05 divided by 1,000,000, typically the number of SNPs tested in a GWAS. We can also view this alternatively as a prior probability that in 10^7 common variants we expect for there to be no more than 10 risk variants for the disease condition. Without a stringent p-value threshold, far too many coincidental false positive associations would be reported.

It is equally important to point out that the p-value threshold of $0.05/1,000,000 = 5 \times 10^{-8}$ does not change no matter how many SNPs are actually tested experimentally in a GWAS. This can be 1,000,000, 100, or even 1 SNP being tested in the case-control populations. For example, at an SNP locus, the two alleles are A/C, with the minor allele C at a frequency > 5%. We ask the question if there is a biased, i.e., associated distribution of the A and C alleles among the control and disease subjects. When the results come back with a $p < 0.05$ for an A-normal and C-disease distribution, should this be considered a genetic association? Or could it be that the biased, associated distribution is completely by accident in the population tested? In the SNP sites that were not tested, how many could by accident have such a biased, associated distribution? The answer is very clear — any of them could. Not testing any of them must not take the stringency away from the one being tested. In genetic association tests, it is still favorable to have a large sample size of case-control subjects, especially when the effect size of the disease variant is small.

Several SNPs in or around the *PRSS8* gene have been reported to be associated with preeclampsia or essential hypertension. These SNPs are located in the coding and non-coding regions of the prostasin gene with some missense mutations, but at present, it is not clear how they impact the prostasin gene expression or the function of the prostasin protein.

Preeclampsia (PE) describes a group of conditions manifested by high blood pressure, swelling of hands and feet, and protein in the urine during pregnancy. The etiology of PE may involve a shallow invasion of the trophoblast cells into the endometrium of the uterus, resulting in an impaired placental vascular remodeling and vascular bed formation, causing placental hypoxia and ischemia. PE usually starts after 20 weeks of pregnancy and ends when pregnancy is terminated and the placenta is expelled from the uterus. There are 5–7% PE cases of all pregnancies worldwide. In a mouse model where the prostasin gene is constitutively inactivated in the germline, the homozygote mouse embryo stopped developing and died before E14.5 (embryonic day 14.5) due to insufficient maturation and invasion of trophoblast cells into the endometrium, greatly affecting placental vascular remodeling. However, the heterozygote mouse embryos developed to term without notable cellular morphological changes. Therefore, the prostasin gene is haplosufficient in the mouse. Studies on the relationship between prostasin SNPs and diseases in human populations yielded inconsistent results.

In 2008, Zhu and colleagues[38] described several prostasin SNPs in or around the prostasin gene, e.g., rs2855475, rs12597511, rs1549294, and rs1549295. But only rs12597512 may be associated with hypertension. However, the absolute blood pressure differences, both systolic and diastolic, are not much, with only about 2 mmHg in difference as discussed by the authors.

In 2011, Li and colleagues[39] identified 10 genetic variants in the prostasin gene after sequencing all exons and the prostasin promoter region of 94 hypertensive individuals of the Xinjiang Kazakhs population. However, these prostasin variants do not seem to relate to the hypertension status.

In 2014, Luo and colleagues[40] reported that the C allele of rs12597511 is the minor allele in Chinese Han women and is associated with a high risk of developing severe preeclampsia during pregnancy.

A similar result was reported in 2021 by Ejaz and colleagues[41] in Pakistani pregnant women showing that the CC genotype at the rs12597511 locus has a higher frequency in hypertensive pregnant women.

From the data presented in the above studies, p-values less than 0.05 were reported, but it is unclear if stringent statistical corrections were performed as required for a proper genetic association analysis.

In the dbSNP database[42], 2,593 entries were pulled out by the key word "prss8", among them three entries were cited in PubMed[43], i.e., rs12597511 (intron_variant); rs8049043 (synonymous_variant); rs2855475 (upstream_transcript_variant). By "somatic" and "missense" categorization, 34 prostasin SNPs were identified among the 2,593.

In 2020, Holt-Danborg and colleagues[44] functionally analyzed 28 prostasin SNPs with missense mutations using an *in vitro* cell-based co-transfection method. Most of the mutations were indistinguishable from the wild-type prostasin in terms of proteolytically activating the matriptase zymogen, except for the following mutations, C70Y, D232G, D134N, I135T, and R44H. The expression, localization, and/or folding of the prostasin protein variants with these mutations might have been altered and compromised due to the mutated amino acid residues, affecting the protease activity. The 28 prostasin SNPs analyzed in this study matched 7 out of 34 prostasin SNPs in the dbSNP database. No human diseases to date have been directly associated to a changed expression level or function of prostasin.

16.5 Prostate cancer

The first attempt of testing if prostasin can be used as a biomarker in cancer was reported in 2001 by Laribi and colleagues[45]. An assay was developed for amplifying prostasin-specific transcripts in blood samples using reverse transcription-polymerase chain reaction (RT-PCR) for the purpose of assisting early prostate cancer diagnosis. In that study, a 546-bp prostasin PCR product was amplified from 36% (35/96) of peripheral blood samples from patients with prostate cancer. Among them, 26% (18/69) of the blood samples were prostasin-positive in patients with localized adenocarcinoma, and 65% (17/27) of the blood samples were prostasin-positive in patients with metastatic disease. The prostasin PCR products were not identified in any of the 86 blood samples from the controls including 47 healthy individuals, 17 with benign prostate hyperplasia, and 22 non-prostate cancer patients.

However, the clinical application and significance of this method were not pursued further.

16.6 Ovarian cancer

Ovarian cancer is a collection of cancers that originate in the ovary, the fallopian tube, or the peritoneum. Depending on the type of cells that the tumor originates from, there are three main types of ovarian cancer. Epithelial cancer is the most common type of ovarian cancer and accounts for ~90% of the malignant ovarian tumors. Rare types of ovarian cancer include germ cell tumors and stromal tumors[46-48]. Based on the morphology, ovarian cancer cells can be well differentiated (grade 1), moderately differentiated (grade 2), and poorly differentiated (grade 3). According to the International Federation of Gynecology and Obstetrics (FIGO)[49], ovarian cancers are categorized into four stages. Stage 1 has cancer cells limited to the ovaries only. Stage 2 has cancer cells spread within the pelvis. Stage 3 has cancer cells spread into the abdominal cavity or lymph nodes. Stage 4 has cancer cells spread to distant organs such as the liver or lung. Most ovarian cancer cases (~63%) are diagnosed in the late stages (stage 3 or 4) of the disease, by then the tumor cells have metastasized beyond the ovaries and the 5-year survival rate is ~27% but is ~93% for the cases diagnosed in stage 1. Therefore, biomarkers for detection of the early-stage ovarian cancers are much needed for screening, as well as for choosing the proper treatment plans. Currently, the U.S. Food and Drug Administration (FDA) approved only a handful of serum markers for ovarian cancer, and none of them are used for the screening propose, but only for the discrimination of pelvic masses, monitoring treatment, or detection of recurrence after treatment. The serum biomarker CA125, also known as mucin 16 (MUC16), is commonly used clinically as an indicator for monitoring the response of patient to therapy in regard to residual or recurrent cancers. It is not a good marker in early stages of the disease due to the CA125 biomarker's low sensitivity (expression level) and low specificity (other cancers may have elevated CA125 levels).

In 2001, Mok and colleagues[50] were the first to suggest that prostasin may be a potential biomarker for ovarian cancer detection, albeit the low number of cases used was one of the limitations of the study mentioned by the authors. First, they transcriptionally profiled 2,400 known human cDNAs spotted on a slide (MICROMAX™ human cDNA microarray system I, NEN Life Science Products, Inc., Boston, MA) using cDNA probes generated from pooled ovarian cancer cell lines (OVCA420, OVCA433, SKOV3) and from pooled normal human ovarian surface epithelial cells (HOSE17, HOSE636, HOSE642). It was determined that prostasin might be overexpressed in the pooled ovarian cancer cells. This result was verified in 10 individual ovarian cancer cell lines (OVCA3, OVCA420, OVCA429, OVCA432, OVCA433, OVCA633, CAOV3, DOV13, SKOV3, ALST) and 4 individual normal ovarian epithelial cell lines (HOSE697, HOSE713, HOSE726, HOSE730) by means of RT-qPCR. The results were further validated by means of immunohistochemistry in ovarian tumor specimens including two serous borderline ovarian tumors, and six serous ovarian cystadenocarcinomas with different tumor grades. Two normal ovaries were also included. Immunoreactive prostasin was identified in the normal ovarian tissues but a stronger staining was observed in the ovarian cancer cells. Similarly, the level of prostasin in the patients' serum was higher than that in the normal individuals. Thus, prostasin was suggested as a potential biomarker for early-stage ovarian cancer detection.

In 2004, Lu and colleagues[51] performed a gene expression analysis and focused on searching for biomarkers for early detection of epithelial ovarian cancer with different histological subtypes. Altogether 42 ovarian carcinoma tumor tissues were analysed, including four histological subtypes (serous, endometrioid, clear cell, and mucinous), I–IV stages, and 1–3 grades of ovarian cancers. Eighty-six genes were identified with at least a 3-fold up-regulation in ovarian cancers when compared with normal epithelial tissues. The prostasin gene was not among the 86. In fact, the prostasin gene expression showed no apparent change in 41 out of 42 cases. The two studies described above relied on different techniques and were performed on specimens recruited at different institutions. These may be the confounding factors contributing to the disagreement of the observed prostasin expression status in ovarian cancers. Costa and colleagues[52] in 2009 were the first to use fresh-frozen ovarian epithelial cancer tissue samples for quantification of prostasin expression by means of conventional RT-PCR and quantitative RT-PCR. The sample size was 12, and 11 were shown to express the prostasin mRNA.

In 2011, Yip and colleagues[53] measured the serum levels of 259 molecules from 499 samples by means of a multiplex immunoassay. They identified prostasin as one of the 175 markers dysregulated in ovarian cancer patient blood. In addition, the level of prostasin in the sera of ovarian cancer patients of all stages displayed an upward trend when compared to that of the benign cases. The differences were statistically significant in stage I samples, not stage II where the biomarker is needed for early detection. No difference of serum prostasin level was observed among clear cell, endometrioid, and mucinous subtypes of ovarian cancers, except for the serous and mixed subtypes. Further, the authors selected the top nine most informative biomarkers with area under the curve (AUC) over 0.800 among the 175 dysregulated markers. When the top nine biomarkers, including prostasin, were combined into a single panel for the correlation analysis, the combined nine markers had better sensitivity and specificity, i.e., a better AUC value (0.950) when compared to the OVA1 panel having an AUC value at 0.912. The OVA1 panel is the Food and Drug Administration-cleared (FDA) multi-analyte test which measures the serum levels of five analytes, CA125, transthyretin (prealbumin), apolipoprotein A1, beta2 microglobulin, and transferrin. It is worth noting that this study compared the serum prostasin levels between ovarian cancers and benign cases without including normal healthy subjects.

In 2013, Chen and colleagues[54] performed a study on 120 samples including 80 adenocarcinoma, 30 cystadenoma (mucinous adenoma), and 10 normal tissues. By means of immunohistochemistry, positive prostasin staining was found in 42.5% of adenocarcinoma, 86.7% of cystadenoma, and 100% of normal tissues, suggesting a down-regulated prostasin expression in ovarian adenocarcinoma. In addition, the presence of prostasin in the tumors is inversely related to the tumor grades and stages, and the lymph node metastatic state; but positively related to the overall survival time.

In 2016, in a bioinformatic study, Tamir and colleagues[55] analyzed the Cancer Gene Index (CGI) database of the National Cancer Institute (NCI, NIH, USA) using the BioXM™ platform. Prostasin was identified as one of the major differentially regulated genes in ovarian cancer (OVC) having a high-expression level. In an array analysis of 312 tissues including normal ovary, benign mass, and OVC tissues, the level of the immunoreactive prostasin protein was confirmed to be high in OVC and benign mass, and independent of grade and stage. Further, an in-house prostasin antibody was used to evaluate the prostasin level in sera by means of immunoblotting, and it was shown that the prostasin level is high in the sera of early-stage OVC but not in the normal or benign samples. The authors suggested that prostasin may be used as a biomarker for screening early-stage OVC, but not for differentiating OVC grades and stages. In addition, prostasin may have a limited use in discriminating subtypes of OVC of late stages (3 and 4), as the expression level seemed to be high in the borderline subtype, followed by the level in the serous, clear cell, endometrial, and papillary serous subtypes.

In 2017, Bastani and colleagues[56] evaluated the sensitivity and specificity of several serum biomarkers for discrimination of epithelial ovarian cancers from benign and healthy controls. The prostasin level in the serum is increased in epithelial ovarian cancers when compared to begin tumors and healthy controls with an AUC (area under curve) value of 0.89, but decreased in late-stage ovarian cancers. This study also reported a down-regulation of prostasin in ovary adenocarcinoma and in mucinous adenoma tissues. Consistent with some reports was the positive correlation between the overall survival and the prostasin expression level.

It appears that the prostasin expression level varies during the progression of ovarian cancers. Results reported by researchers are not at all consistent with one another. The factors affecting the results could come from the source of subjects/samples, the database, the method of evaluation, and more important, the choice of prostasin-detecting antibodies, for which the sensitivity and the specificity need to be scrutinized, verified, and normalized.

16.7 Renal cell carcinoma (RCC)

Prostasin expression is found in the chromophobe subtype of RCC but rarely in oncocytoma, a benign neoplasm. Although these two tumors are distinct from each other biologically, there are currently no unequivocal markers to separate them apart. Prostasin may potentially be explored as a biomarker in this case. It was not clear from the study if the level of prostasin expression in the chromophobe tumors is comparable to that in the normal kidney[57].

In general, the prostasin protein expression is usually found to be less in advanced cancers (as discussed in detail in Chapter 14). This makes it intrinsically challenging for biomarker development. The expression level of the prostasin protein in cancer tissues and in bodily fluids were investigated for more than 20 years but with no conclusive results appropriate for consideration of further development toward application as a true biomarker.

16.8 Computer-based prediction

The coronavirus disease 2019 (COVID-19) pandemic is caused by the infection of severe acute respiratory syndrome coronavirus 2 (SARS-CoV-2), a new strain of the beta coronavirus. Laboratory experiments suggested that this virus binds to angiotensin-converting enzyme 2 (ACE2) on the airway cell surface via its Spike (S) protein, a viral surface glycoprotein. The Spike protein is subsequently cleaved by serine proteases furin and TMPRSS2 to enable viral fusion and entry in human airway cells for replication and spread[58–60].

In 2021, Hossain and colleagues[61] carried out an *In Silico* Analysis utilizing the functional conjugation approach and supported this hypothesis while predicating that ACE2, TMPRSS2, and furin are functionally co-dependent of one another. In addition, an analysis using SEEK (Search-based Exploration of Expression Kompendia) identified *PRSS8* (prostasin) as commonly co-expressed with *ACE2*, *TMPRSS2*, and *FURIN*, but no functional interactions have been established so far for prostasin with the other enzymes.

In 2021, Gao and colleagues[62] analyzed the miRNA and gene expression profiles of patients with idiopathic pulmonary fibrosis (IPF) using the Gene Expression Omnibus database. Prostasin expression was found to be down-regulated in IPF.

16.9 Drug targets and therapeutics

In 2013, Rowe and colleagues[63] performed a proof-of-concept pilot study assessing the feasibility of a nasal spray with the serine protease inhibitor camostat to treat cystic fibrosis (CF) patients with an intent of attenuating the airway ENaC activity by inhibiting the prostasin activity. Although intranasal administration of camostat inhibited the ENaC activity, the specificity of camostat to the prostasin serine protease requires further investigation because camostat can inhibit other serine proteases to reduce the ENaC activity.

In 2021, Xu and colleagues[64] assembled a genomic-based gene lists containing several genes known for an association with the late-onset Alzheimer's disease (AD). Clinical AD drugs were then applied to the gene list to find potential candidate drugs with the help of a computational program. Interestingly, prostasin was identified as a drug target of Alzheimer's disease (AD).

References

1. Yu JX, Chao L, Chao J (1994). Prostasin is a novel human serine proteinase from seminal fluid. Purification, tissue distribution, and localization in prostate gland. *J Biol Chem.* 269(29):18843–18848.
2. Narikiyo T, Kitamura K, Adachi M, Miyoshi T, Iwashita K, Shiraishi N, Nonoguchi H, Chen LM, Chai KX, Chao J, Tomita K (2002). Regulation of prostasin by aldosterone in the kidney. *J Clin Invest.* 109(3): 401–408.
3. Olivieri O, Castagna A, Guarini P, Chiecchi L, Sabaini G, Pizzolo F, Corrocher R, Righetti PG (2005). Urinary prostasin: A candidate marker of epithelial sodium channel activation in humans. *Hypertension.* 46(4):683–688.

4. Koda A, Wakida N, Toriyama K, Yamamoto K, Iijima H, Tomita K, Kitamura K (2009). Urinary prostasin in humans: Relationships among prostasin, aldosterone and epithelial sodium channel activity. *Hypertens Res.* 32(4):276–281.

5. Zhu H, Chao J, Guo D, Li K, Huang Y, Hawkins K, Wright N, Stallmann-Jorgensen I, Yan W, Harshfield GA, Dong Y (2009). Urinary prostasin: A possible biomarker for renal pressure natriuresis in black adolescents. *Pediatr Res.* 65(4):443–446.

6. Olivieri O, Chiecchi L, Pizzolo F, Castagna A, Raffaelli R, Gunasekaran M, Guarini P, Consoli L, Salvagno G, Kitamura K (2013). Urinary prostasin in normotensive individuals: Correlation with the aldosterone to renin ratio and urinary sodium. *Hypertens Res.* 36(6):528–533.

7. Guo DH, Parikh SJ, Chao J, Pollock NK, Wang X, Snieder H, Navis G, Wilson JG, Bhagatwala J, Zhu H, Dong Y (2013). Urinary prostasin excretion is associated with adiposity in nonhypertensive African-American adolescents. *Pediatr Res.* 74(2):206–210.

8. Andersen H, Friis UG, Hansen PB, Svenningsen P, Henriksen JE, Jensen BL (2015). Diabetic nephropathy is associated with increased urine excretion of proteases plasmin, prostasin and urokinase and activation of amiloride-sensitive current in collecting duct cells. *Nephrol Dial Transplant.* 30(5):781–789.

9. Frederiksen-Møller B, Jørgensen JS, Hansen MR, Krigslund O, Vogel LK, Andersen LB, Jensen BL (2016). Prostasin and matriptase (ST14) in placenta from preeclamptic and healthy pregnant women. *J Hypertens.* 34(2):298–306.

10. Zheng H, Liu X, Sharma NM, Li Y, Pliquett RU, Patel KP (2016). Urinary proteolytic activation of renal epithelial Na+ channels in chronic heart failure. *Hypertension.* 67(1):197–205.

11. Pizzolo F, Chiecchi L, Morandini F, Castagna A, Zorzi F, Zaltron C, Pattini P, Chiariello C, Salvagno G, Olivieri O (2017). Increased urinary excretion of the epithelial Na channel activator prostasin in patients with primary aldosteronism. *J Hypertens.* 35(2):355–361.

12. Oxlund C, Kurt B, Schwarzensteiner I, Hansen MR, Stæhr M, Svenningsen P, Jacobsen IA, Hansen PB, Thuesen AD, Toft A, Hinrichs GR, Bistrup C, Jensen BL (2017). Albuminuria is associated with an increased prostasin in urine while aldosterone has no direct effect on urine and kidney tissue abundance of prostasin. *Pflugers Arch.* 469(5–6): 655–667.

13. Hinrichs GR, Michelsen JS, Zachar R, Friis UG, Svenningsen P, Birn H, Bistrup C, Jensen BL (2018). Albuminuria in kidney transplant recipients is associated with increased urinary serine proteases and activation of the epithelial sodium channel. *Am J Physiol Renal Physiol.* 315(1):F151–F160.

14. Raghu G, Richeldi L, Jagerschmidt A, Martin V, Subramaniam A, Ozoux ML, Esperet CA, Soubrane C (2018). Idiopathic pulmonary fibrosis: Prospective, case-controlled study of natural history and circulating biomarkers. *Chest.* 154(6):1359–1370.

15. Lal C, Hardiman G, Kumbhare S, Strange C (2019). Proteomic biomarkers of cognitive impairment in obstructive sleep apnea syndrome. *Sleep Breath.* 23(1):251–257.

16. Stattin K, Lind L, Elmståhl S, Wolk A, Lemming EW, Melhus H, Michaëlsson K, Byberg L (2019). Physical activity is associated with a large number of cardiovascular-specific proteins: Cross-sectional analyses in two independent cohorts. *Eur J Prev Cardiol.* 26(17):1865–1873.

17. Pietzner M, Wheeler E, Carrasco-Zanini J, Cortes A, Koprulu M, Wörheide MA, Oerton E, Cook J, Stewart ID, Kerrison ND, Luan J, Raffler J, Arnold M, Arlt W, O'Rahilly S, Kastenmüller G, Gamazon ER, Hingorani AD, Scott RA, Wareham NJ, Langenberg C (2021). Mapping the proteo-genomic convergence of human diseases. *Science.* 374(6569):eabj1541.

18. Dunlay SM, Roger VL, Redfield MM (2017). Epidemiology of heart failure with preserved ejection fraction. *Nat Rev Cardiol.* 14(10): 591–602.

19. Edelmann F, Schmidt AG, Gelbrich G, Binder L, Herrmann-Lingen C, Halle M, Hasenfuss G, Wachter R, Pieske B (2010). Rationale and design of the 'aldosterone receptor blockade in diastolic heart failure' trial: A double-blind, randomized, placebo-controlled, parallel group study to determine the effects of spironolactone on exercise capacity and diastolic function in patients with symptomatic diastolic heart failure (Aldo-DHF). *Eur J Heart Fail.* 12(8):874–882.

20. Edelmann F, Wachter R, Schmidt AG, Kraigher-Krainer E, Colantonio C, Kamke W, Duvinage A, Stahrenberg R, Durstewitz K, Löffler M, Düngen HD, Tschöpe C, Herrmann-Lingen C, Halle M, Hasenfuss G, Gelbrich G, Pieske B, Aldo-DHF Investigators (2013). Effect of spironolactone on diastolic function and exercise capacity in patients with

heart failure with preserved ejection fraction: The Aldo-DHF random-ized controlled trial. *JAMA.* 309(8):781–791.

21. Schnelle M, Leha A, Eidizadeh A, Fuhlrott K, Trippel TD, Hashemi D, Toischer K, Wachter R, Herrmann-Lingen C, Hasenfuß G, Pieske B, Binder L, Edelmann F (2021). Plasma biomarker profiling in heart failure patients with preserved ejection fraction before and after spirono-lactone treatment: Results from the Aldo-DHF trial. *Cells.* 10(10):2796.

22. Cauwenberghs N, Sabovčik F, Magnus A, Haddad F, Kuznetsova T (2021). Proteomic profiling for detection of early-stage heart failure in the community. *ESC Heart Fail.* 8(4):2928–2939.

23. Verdonschot JAJ, Ferreira JP, Pellicori P, Brunner-La Rocca HP, Clark AL, Cosmi F, Cuthbert J, Girerd N, Mariottoni B, Petutschnigg J, Ros-signol P, Cleland JGF, Zannad F, Heymans SRB, HOMAGE "Heart Omics in AGEing" consortium (2021). Proteomic mechanistic profile of patients with diabetes at risk of developing heart failure: Insights from the HOMAGE trial. *Cardiovasc Diabetol.* 20(1):163.

24. Jacobs L, Thijs L, Jin Y, Zannad F, Mebazaa A, Rouet P, Pinet F, Bauters C, Pieske B, Tomaschitz A, Mamas M, Diez J, McDonald K, Cleland JG, Brunner-La Rocca HP, Heymans S, Latini R, Masson S, Sever P, Delles C, Pocock S, Collier T, Kuznetsova T, Staessen JA (2014). Heart 'omics' in AGEing (HOMAGE): Design, research objectives and characteristics of the common database. *J Biomed Res.* 28(5):349–359.

25. Chandramouli C, Ting TW, Tromp J, Agarwal A, Svedlund S, Saraste A, Hage C, Tan RS, Beussink-Nelson L, Lagerström Fermer M, Gan LM, Lund L, Shah SJ, Lam CSP (2022). Sex differences in proteomic cor-relates of coronary microvascular dysfunction among patients with heart failure and preserved ejection fraction. *Eur J Heart Fail.* 24(4):681–684.

26. Sekine T, Takizawa S, Uchimura K, Miyazaki A, Tsuchiya K (2021). Liver-specific overexpression of prostasin attenuates high-fat diet-induced metabolic dysregulation in mice. *Int J Mol Sci.* 22(15):8314.

27. Uchimura K, Hayata M, Mizumoto T, Miyasato Y, Kakizoe Y, Morinaga J, Onoue T, Yamazoe R, Ueda M, Adachi M, Miyoshi T, Shiraishi N, Ogawa W, Fukuda K, Kondo T, Matsumura T, Araki E, Tomita K, Kit-amura K (2014). The serine protease prostasin regulates hepatic insulin sensitivity by modulating TLR4 signalling. *Nat Commun.* 5:3428.

28. Bao X, Xu B, Muhammad IF, Nilsson PM, Nilsson J, Engström G (2022). Plasma prostasin: A novel risk marker for incidence of diabetes and cancer mortality. *Diabetologia.* 65(10):1642–1651.

29. Doyle LM, Wang MZ (2019). Overview of extracellular vesicles, their origin, composition, purpose, and methods for exosome isolation and analysis. *Cells.* 8(7):727.

30. van der Lubbe N, Jansen PM, Salih M, Fenton RA, van den Meiracker AH, Danser AH, Zietse R, Hoorn EJ (2012). The phosphorylated sodium chloride cotransporter in urinary exosomes is superior to prostasin as a marker for aldosteronism. *Hypertension.* 60(3):741–748.

31. Castagna A, Pizzolo F, Chiecchi L, Morandini F, Channavajjhala SK, Guarini P, Salvagno G, Olivieri O (2015). Circadian exosomal expression of renal thiazide-sensitive NaCl cotransporter (NCC) and prostasin in healthy individuals. *Proteomics Clin Appl.* 9(5–6):623–639.

32. Bartter FC, Delea CS (1962). A map of blood and urinary changes related to circadian variations in adrenal cortical function in normal subjects. *Ann N Y Acad Sci.* 98:969–983.

33. Qi Y, Wang X, Rose KL, MacDonald WH, Zhang B, Schey KL, Luther JM (2016). Activation of the endogenous renin-angiotensin-aldosterone system or aldosterone administration increases urinary exosomal sodium channel excretion. *J Am Soc Nephrol.* 27(2):646–656.

34. Zachar R, Jensen BL, Svenningsen P (2019). Dietary Na+ intake in healthy humans changes the urine extracellular vesicle prostasin abundance while the vesicle excretion rate, NCC, and ENaC are not altered. *Am J Physiol Renal Physiol.* 317(6):F1612–F1622.

35. Krishnamachary B, Cook C, Spikes L, Chalise P, Dhillon NK (2020). The potential role of extracellular vesicles in COVID-19 associated endothelial injury and pro-inflammation. *medRxiv* [Preprint]. PMID: 32909001.

36. Fontana S, Mauceri R, Novara ME, Alessandro R, Campisi G (2021). Protein cargo of salivary small extracellular vesicles as potential functional signature of oral squamous cell carcinoma. *Int J Mol Sci.* 22(20):11160.

37. Birn H, Christensen EI (2006). Renal albumin absorption in physiology and pathology. *Kidney Int.* 69(3):440–449.

38. Zhu H, Guo D, Li K, Yan W, Tan Y, Wang X, Treiber FA, Chao J, Snieder H, Dong Y (2008). Prostasin: A possible candidate gene for human hypertension. *Am J Hypertens.* 21(9):1028–1033.

39. Li NF, Zhang JH, Chang JH, Yang J, Wang HM, Zhou L, Luo WL (2011). Association of genetic variations of the prostasin gene with essential hypertension in the Xinjiang Kazakh population. *Chin Med J (Engl).* 124(14):2107–2112.

40. Luo D, Zhang Y, Bai Y, Liu X, Gong Y, Zhou B, Zhang L, Luo L, Zhou R (2014). Prostasin gene polymorphism at rs12597511 is associated with severe preeclampsia in Chinese Han women. *Chin Med J (Engl)*. 127(11):2048–2052.
41. Ejaz S, Ali A, Riffat S, Mahmood A, Azim K (2021). Genetic polymorphism of the prostasin gene in hypertensive pregnant Pakistani females. *Pak J Med Sci*. 37(1):109–113.
42. dbSNP database (https://www.ncbi.nlm.nih.gov/snp/)
43. PubMed (https://pubmed.ncbi.nlm.nih.gov)
44. Holt-Danborg L, Skovbjerg S, Goderum KW, Nonboe AW, Stankevic E, Frost ÁK, Vitved L, Jensen JK, Vogel LK (2020). Insights into the regulation of the matriptase-prostasin proteolytic system. *Biochem J*. 477(22):4349–4365.
45. Laribi A, Berteau P, Gala J, Eschwège P, Benoit G, Tombal B, Schmitt F, Loric S (2001). Blood-borne RT-PCR assay for prostasin-specific transcripts to identify circulating prostate cells in cancer patients. *Eur Urol*. 39(1):65–71.
46. Chen VW, Ruiz B, Killeen JL, Coté TR, Wu XC, Correa CN (2003). Pathology and classification of ovarian tumors. *Cancer*. 97(10 Suppl):2631–2642.
47. Algeciras-Schimnich A (2013). A review of current serum markers and their clinical applications. *Clinical Laboratory News*.
48. Matz M, Coleman MP, Sant M, Chirlaque MD, Visser O, Gore M, Allemani C; & the CONCORD Working Group (2017). The histology of ovarian cancer: Worldwide distribution and implications for international survival comparisons (CONCORD-2). *Gynecol Oncol*. 144(2):405–413.
49. International Federation of Gynecology and Obstetrics (FIGO).
50. Mok SC, Chao J, Skates S, Wong K, Yiu GK, Muto MG, Berkowitz RS, Cramer DW (2001). Prostasin, a potential serum marker for ovarian cancer: Identification through microarray technology. *J Natl Cancer Inst*. 93(19):1458–1464.
51. Lu KH, Patterson AP, Wang L, Marquez RT, Atkinson EN, Baggerly KA, Ramoth LR, Rosen DG, Liu J, Hellstrom I, Smith D, Hartmann L, Fishman D, Berchuck A, Schmandt R, Whitaker R, Gershenson DM, Mills GB, Bast RC Jr (2004). Selection of potential markers for epithelial ovarian cancer with gene expression arrays and recursive descent partition analysis. *Clin Cancer Res*. 10(10):3291–3300.
52. Costa FP, Batista EL Jr, Zelmanowicz A, Svedman C, Devenz G, Alves S, Silva AS, Garicochea B (2009). Prostasin, a potential tumor marker in ovarian cancer-a pilot study. *Clinics (Sao Paulo)*. 64(7):641–644.

53. Yip P, Chen TH, Seshaiah P, Stephen LL, Michael-Ballard KL, Mapes JP, Mansheld BC, Bertenshaw CP (2011) Comprehensive serum profiling for the discovery of epithelial ovarian cancer biomarkers. *PLoS One.* 6(12):e29533.

54. Chen PX, Li QY, Yang Z (2013). Axl and prostasin are biomarkers for prognosis of ovarian adenocarcinoma. *Ann Diagn Pathol.* 17(5): 425–429.

55. Tamir A, Gangadharan A, Balwani S, Tanaka T, Patel U, Hassan A, Benke S, Agas A, D'Agostino J, Shin D, Yoon S, Goy A, Pecora A, Suh KS (2016). The serine protease prostasin (PRSS8) is a potential biomarker for early detection of ovarian cancer. *J Ovarian Res.* 9:20.

56. Bastani A, Asghary A, Heidari MH, Karimi-Busheri F (2017). Evaluation of the sensitivity and specificity of serum level of prostasin, CA125, LDH, AFP, and hCG+β in epithelial ovarian cancer patients. *Eur J Gynaecol Oncol.* 38(3):418–424.

57. Rohan S, Tu JJ, Kao J, Mukherjee P, Campagne F, Zhou XK, Hyjek E, Alonso MA, Chen YT (2006). Gene expression profiling separates chromophobe renal cell carcinoma from oncocytoma and identifies vesicular transport and cell junction proteins as differentially expressed genes. *Clin Cancer Res.* 12(23):6937–6945.

58. Li W, Moore MJ, Vasilieva N, Sui J, Wong SK, Berne MA, Somasundaran M, Sullivan JL, Luzuriaga K, Greenough TC, Choe H, Farzan M (2003). Angiotensin-converting enzyme 2 is a functional receptor for the SARS coronavirus. *Nature.* 426(6965):450–454.

59. Shulla A, Heald-Sargent T, Subramanya G, Zhao J, Perlman S, Gallagher T (2011). A transmembrane serine protease is linked to the severe acute respiratory syndrome coronavirus receptor and activates virus entry. *J Virol.* 85(2):873–882.

60. Hoffmann M, Kleine-Weber H, Schroeder S, Krüger N, Herrler T, Erichsen S, Schiergens TS, Herrler G, Wu NH, Nitsche A, Müller MA, Drosten C, Pöhlmann S (2020). SARS-CoV-2 1pends on ACE2 and TMPRSS2 and is blocked by a clinically proven protease inhibitor. *Cell.* 181(2):271–280.e8.

61. Hossain MS, Tonmoy MIQ, Fariha A, Islam MS, Roy AS, Islam MN, Kar K, Alam MR, Rahaman MM (2021). Prediction of the effects of variants and differential expression of key host genes ACE2, TMPRSS2, and FURIN in SARS-CoV-2 pathogenesis: An in silico approach. *Bioinform Biol Insights.* 15:11779322211054684.

62. Gao L, Li P, Tian H, Wu M, Yang J, Xu X (2021). Screening of biomarkers involved in idiopathic pulmonary fibrosis and regulation of upstream miRNAs. *Am J Med Sci.* 363(1):55–63.

63. Rowe SM, Reeves G, Hathorne H, Solomon GM, Abbi S, Renard D, Lock R, Zhou P, Danahay H, Clancy JP, Waltz DA (2013). Reduced sodium transport with nasal administration of the prostasin inhibitor camostat in subjects with cystic fibrosis. *Chest.* 144(1):200–207.

64. Xu Y, Kong J, Hu P (2021). Computational drug repurposing for alzheimer's disease using risk genes from GWAS and single-cell RNA sequencing studies. *Front Pharmacol.* 12:617537.

Epilogue

How important is prostasin? Prostasin may have originated and derived from bony vertebrates over 435 million years ago (Mya) and the gene tree is conserved since the tetrapods about 351 Mya. We have highlighted the work that assigned an orthologue with a functional role in the blood coagulation for prostasin in the zebrafish, evolved from about 400 Mya. That says how important prostasin is and how much prostasin is required along the long history of speciation. From what we have learned so far, what matters the most is the physical and the structural presence of the prostasin protein in a cell, a tissue, an organ, and the body in a spatially and temporally regulated state. The structure dictates but also informs on the function.

To begin, in the mouse, an egg does not have prostasin, but a sperm does. Once fertilized, the zygote requires prostasin to invade into the uterus to seek a shelter and to develop a placenta from which the developing embryo gets the nutrients to support and sustain life. Without prostasin, the placenta can be formed but with impaired functions and will not support the embryo to develop to term. The embryos without prostasin die in utero within 14.5 days of gestation. Interestingly, prostasin is not required for the embryos to grow to term when they are inside the amniotic sac. Once born, the neonatal skin requires prostasin to develop and mature. Otherwise, mice without prostasin in the skin will die within 60 hours as a result of dehydration. There are currently no known diseases identified with a genetic defect in the prostasin gene.

Is prostasin required for the adult life? The lack of a genetic association with a disease can be interpreted in two ways. One, prostasin is somewhat dispensable. We have seen in the research finding highlights that some functions performed by prostasin can be compensated by redundant systems or molecules. Many genetic variants have been reported for the prostasin gene locus but there is no disease association. Clearly not all such variants have been investigated for a potential functional alteration, and some may be expected to have such an impact. Alternatively, any variant that results in a total loss of prostasin function may not be tolerated and would be lost in reproduction, or a lack thereof.

The lesser impactful variants and the variations of prostasin expression in the adult life can make the conditions less than ideal for the relevant tissues and organs, thus affecting the adult life in many ways. In the lung, prostasin functions to remove the excess water out of the airways to enable air exchange. In the skin, prostasin functions to retain the water to keep the skin moisturized. In the kidney, prostasin regulates water and Na^+ reabsorption to maintain the proper extracellular fluid volume. In the colon, prostasin maintains immune tolerance and reduces inflammation via toll-like receptor 4 (TLR4). In the prostate, prostasin in the prostasomes in the seminal plasma may be a mechanism employed for sperm protection such as immune tolerance. In the bladder, prostasin maintains the urothelial cells in the differentiated state in concert with E-cadherin. When prostasin is absent in the lung, kidney, and colon, the adult life is not immediately upset to an extreme degree because there may be compensatory pathways and mechanisms that kick in to maintain the bodily functions at a manageable status, if no other insult is compounded. Under such a challenge however, either acute or chronic, such as an infection or aging, immediate and chronic conditions will develop to "highlight" the prostasin defect.

Genetically, the prostasin locus is described to be haplosufficient, literally "half is enough", thus some potential loss-of-function variants can be tolerated in the heterozygote state. Only when the prostasin expression level or its function is reduced by at least more than half of the full capacity, or the strengths of the challenge surpass the compensatory capability, should prostasin-related pathological conditions or diseases begin to develop and evolve. The human prostasin gene is epigenetically regulated through promoter DNA methylation and histone modifications. This mechanism makes prostasin expression responsive to both acute and chronic changes in the cellular and physiological environments. Acute factors may be either external or internal, such as pathogens or hormones, while dietary habits and aging itself are chronic factors. The "epigenetic clock" is a measurement of aging based on the chemical modification changes of biomolecules especially the DNA methylation changes in various tissues and organs. The epigenetic clock on the prostasin gene and how its expression changes over the course of aging in various parts of the body have not been investigated. For such an important protein, no diseases are currently assigned to prostasin variants or defects but a limited scope of genetic phenotypic association studies implicated the prostasin locus in an aging-related disease, Alzheimer's. The fact that epithelial cancers, a disease also associated with aging, typically show a down-regulation to absence of prostasin expression with progression, should be considered a very good reason to look at its epigenetic clock. The past research laid a solid foundation for future endeavors to uncover the critical clues to guide us in maintaining our "prostasin health" through lifestyle or medicinal interventions.

Many thanks go to all the researchers who published and shared their data and thoughts on prostasin's functions, which are still somewhat of a terra incognita — ever since its discovery in the laboratory of Dr. Julie Chao, with her graduate student Jack Yu in 1993.

The author is humbled by this opportunity to write about prostasin, and appreciates the support from Dr. Karl Chai on completing this book, especially his editing of the text language, as well as his constructive suggestions on the figure illustrations and the contents.

Index

16p11.2, 27, 35–37, 53

albuminuria, 206, 213
aldosterone, 65, 66, 74–76,
    78–80, 87, 102, 103, 183, 184,
    194, 204–206, 208, 209,
    212
allele, 22, 68, 70, 103, 150,
    214–216
Alzheimer's, 37, 209, 223, 233
amiloride 54, 75–77, 102, 103,
    194, 195, 205, 206
aprotinin, 23–25, 42, 52, 75, 88,
    121, 190, 206
ASL (airway surface liquid), 85,
    86, 88, 90–93, 184

biomarker, vi, viii, 16, 166, 203,
    204, 207, 209, 210, 211, 213,
    217–222
Bonferroni, 211, 215

cadherin, 93, 100, 163–165, 171,
    172, 232
cancer,
    bladder, 161, 163–165

breast, 70, 159–161, 164–166,
    187
cervical, 169
colon, 165, 167, 168, 170
definition, 157
esophagus, 161, 165, 171
gastric, 161, 169
glioma, 172, 173
liver, 170, 171
lung, 149, 165, 172
oral, 165, 173, 174, 213
ovarian, 147, 165–167,
    218–221
prostate, 80, 145, 159–162,
    164, 165, 184, 185, 207, 208,
    217
CAP1 (channel-activating protease
    1), 32, 79, 125, 126
cascade, 1, 6, 7, 13, 14, 57, 116,
    139, 146, 184, 187, 194
CSD (congenital sodium diarrhea),
    104, 105, 191
CTE (congenital tufting
    enteropathy), 104, 105
cystic fibrosis, 32, 86, 90–93, 195,
    223

diabetes, 151, 152, 206–208, 210, 211

diet, 69, 102, 103, 141, 151, 152, 168, 184, 189, 195, 204, 212

differentiation, xii, 11, 58, 99, 100, 105, 111, 114–117, 123, 125, 127, 128, 134, 136, 138, 164, 165, 171, 174

EGFR (epidermal growth factor receptor), 93, 126, 128, 134, 172, 184

egg, xi, xii, 121, 129, 231

embryo, xi, xii, 65, 67–69, 122, 123, 124, 126, 127, 129, 163, 216, 231

EMT, vii, 163, 165, 168, 172

epcam (epithelial cell adhesion molecule), 104–107

epidermis, 58, 66, 69, 85, 111–115, 117

epigenetic, xiii, 49, 70, 107, 129, 141, 160, 161, 203, 233

exosomes, viii, 16, 80, 121, 148, 149, 158, 172, 175, 203, 206, 212

genetics, vii, 21, 27, 29, 31, 32, 58, 146, 152

gestation, 113, 123, 124, 231

GPI (glycosylphosphatidylinositol), 13–16, 28, 41, 42, 51–55, 58, 76–78

GWAS (genome-wide metaanalysis), 37, 152, 153, 209, 214, 215

hai-1 (hepatocyte growth factor activator inhibitor 1), 4–6, 57, 116, 124, 190–192

hai-2 (hepatocyte growth factor activator inhibitor 2), 4, 57, 105–107, 116, 124, 174, 190–192

histone, xii, 37, 38, 41, 70, 160, 161, 164, 169, 203, 233

IBD (inflammatory bowel disease), 99, 140

ifn (interferon), 67, 135, 137, 172

innate, 68, 108, 111, 133, 134, 136, 140, 142, 186

interstitial, viii, 86, 208

irreversible, 4, 6, 57, 193

junction, vii, viii, 99, 100, 101, 104–106, 113, 114, 116, 127, 128, 137, 139, 141, 158, 163, 183, 192

kat8 (K (lysine) acetyltransferase 8), 37, 40, 41, 209

LPS (lipopolysaccharide), 67, 68, 134–141, 151, 186

methylation, xii, 38, 160, 161, 164, 169, 203, 232, 233

modification, xii, xiii, 6, 14, 32, 38, 76, 92, 151, 160, 185, 203, 233

OMIM (Online Mendelian
Inheritance in Man), 37, 63, 65,
68, 147
oxyanion, 1, 2, 49, 56, 182,
194

PAR-2, vii, 185, 186
PD-L1, 137, 172
permeability, vii, 101–103, 106,
113, 114, 137, 141, 168
phospholipase, 15, 16, 53, 121,
203
placebo, 206, 208
placenta, viii, 68, 122, 123, 125,
126–128, 139, 145, 149, 188,
190, 216, 231
PN-1 (protease nexin-1), 4, 57,
124, 182, 193, 194
preeclampsia, 123, 127, 205, 208,
215, 216
proliferation, vii, viii, 11, 12, 58,
70, 100, 105, 111, 113–116,
123, 125–128, 160, 164, 167,
170, 171, 173, 174
promoter, 38, 43, 67, 69, 103,
126, 127, 136, 138, 150–152,
160–162, 164, 169, 189, 203,
216, 232

reversible, 4, 6, 29, 42, 57, 75,
107, 124, 141, 181, 189
RNA
miRNA, 163, 170
lncRNA, 169, 170
siRNA, 93, 194
RTK (receptor tyrosine kinase), vii,
54, 57, 142, 184

sensitivity, 206, 218, 220, 221
serpin (serine protease inhibitor),
25, 31, 57, 189, 193
slug, 13, 38, 138, 13, 38,
162–165
snail, 163, 171
SNP (single-nucleotide
polymorphism), 37, 104, 105,
214–217
specificity, 5, 15, 16, 23, 43, 51,
55, 190, 211, 218, 220, 221,
223
sperm, xi, xii, 41, 55, 115, 121,
129, 231, 232
spironolactone, 204, 206–211
SREBP (stero-regulatory
element-binding protein), 38,
152, 162, 163, 203

TGF (transforming growth factor),
123
therapeutic, vi, viii, 92, 94, 107,
128, 174, 203, 223
TLR4 (toll-like receptor 4), 57,
68, 134, 135, 137, 139–142,
151, 152, 186
TMPRSS, 186
TMPRSS1, 54
TMPRSS2, 87, 88, 134, 195,
222
TMPRSS13, 54, 186, 187
tolerance, viii, 69, 128, 232
tPA (tissue plasminogen activator),
8, 123
trait, 21, 36, 152, 153, 209
trophoblast, 122–128, 139, 188,
216

uPA (urokinase-type plasminogen
   activator), 8, 123
urinary, 22, 75, 79, 103, 127, 134,
   149, 158, 194, 195, 204–208,
   212, 213
uterus, 39, 40, 121, 122, 128,
   145, 216, 231

validation, 32, 211, 213

X-ray, 50, 51, 54, 182

zygote, 122, 128, 129, 231
zymogen, 6, 13, 51, 56, 58, 115,
   116, 146, 148, 185, 187–189, 217

CPSIA information can be obtained
at www.ICGtesting.com
Printed in the USA
BVHW050932090323
659800BV00002B/61